THE TREATMENT OF THE
CHILD AT HOME
A GUIDE FOR FAMILY DOCTORS

The Treatment of the Child at Home

a guide for family doctors

R. S. ILLINGWORTH

M.D. F.R.C.P. D.P.H. D.C.H.

Professor of Child Health
The University of Sheffield

Blackwell Scientific Publications
Oxford and Edinburgh

© 1971 by Blackwell Scientific Publications
5 Alfred Street, Oxford, England and
9 Forrest Road, Edinburgh, Scotland

All rights reserved. No part of this publication
may be reproduced, stored in a retrieval system,
or transmitted, in any form or by any means,
electronic, mechanical, photocopying, recording
or otherwise without the prior permission of
the copyright owner.

ISBN 0 632 08400 6

First published 1971

Distributed in the USA by
F. A. Davis Company, 1915 Arch Street,
Philadelphia, Pennsylvania

Printed in Great Britain by
Western Printing Services Ltd.
Bristol
and bound by
The Kemp Hall Bindery, Oxford

Contents

Appendixes

Preface

This book is intended for the family doctor. It was written because, so far as I know, there is no book for him about the treatment of the child in the home. There are excellent books on paediatric therapeutics (such as those of Shirkey, Kagan and Gellis) but they are too big for the family doctor because they include treatment which can or should be carried out only in hospital. The needs of the family doctor are quite different from those of the hospital doctor, and in this book I have purposely excluded treatments which should be given only by the hospital consultant or his assistants. Obviously the question of what should and should not be treated in the home is a matter of opinion, and is to some extent governed by the family doctor's interests, experience and facilities; but in this book I have throughout expressed my own view as to the conditions and circumstances for which I think that hospital or specialist consultation or treatment is advisable.

Although the book is intended for the family doctor, I hope that medical students and junior hospital doctors will find it useful, as it discusses common conditions which are treated at home or in the out-patient department; but it definitely does not provide all that they need to know about treatment, since treatment which should or can be given only in hospital has been rigorously excluded.

My aim has been to keep the book brief and practical, avoiding long lists of possible drugs and treatments, and confining it to the treatment which I personally recommend, naming alternatives if relevant. There is a current textbook of therapeutics which lists 28 drugs for the treatment of epilepsy. I feel that such a list would merely confuse a family doctor. My choices of treatment are clearly open to criticism, for in numerous conditions there is no one treatment. All doctors have their therapeutic preferences, and in this book I have presented mine – and am prepared to defend them. No one is an expert in everything, and I have drawn heavily on the experience of my colleagues. My experience of general practice is limited and was gained many years ago; but continued experience in a busy out-patient department is a constant reminder of the problems of the family doctor in the home.

In therapeutics there is little place for dogma. For example, an ammonia dermatitis nappy rash will respond to many different treatments. No one has conducted a controlled trial in order to decide between them, so that any statement as to which is the best treatment can only be based on clinical impression. Similarly with infant foods; it would be unscientific to declare firmly that any one food is better than another – though we can certainly say that some foods have the advantage over others in price. One cannot prove everything, nor is it worth trying to do so. For instance, no one has conducted a trial of the numerous different antihistamines or corticosteroid ointments and creams (numbering over 90); unless proper clinical trials have been conducted, no one should state categorically that any one is better than another.

My opinion is based on evidence, if there is any; otherwise on clinical impression and experience. I have always tried to profit from experience by following up patients whom I treat; but it would be a serious mistake to assume that the doctor with the most experience is the best qualified to be dogmatic about treatment. Many doctors, as they grow older and more experienced, merely repeat the same mistakes with increasing confidence. I shall repeat constantly that if one is to learn and if one is to do one's best for one's patients, a proper follow-up is essential. In my opinion the commonest mistake in treatment is over-confidence with resulting failure to follow up in order to determine the response to treatment.

I have emphasized throughout that one must treat the whole child, and not merely the presenting symptom. The family doctor is in an ideal position to understand the personal and parental background of the child's symptoms and to try to help the child in the light of this knowledge. If he fails to treat the psychological factors in a child's illness, or merely prescribes drugs as a substitute for counselling the parents with regard to the child's behaviour, he will fail his patient. On innumerable occasions the good family doctor, when asked to advise about a child's symptoms, will not prescribe any medicines whether there is disease or not. The good doctor must know not only when to treat, but when not to treat. If no drug or treatment is required, I have said so clearly; but I have constantly borne in mind some words of Sir Francis Walshe in another connection: 'This is scientific nihilism, disguised as its opposite, scientific logic and precision.' I have tried to avoid therapeutic nihilism.

Almost all drugs have possible side effects, and I have reproduced a section on side effects of drugs from my book, *Common Symptoms of Disease in Children*. I have made numerous references to that book, because this book is in a way complementary to it. Proper treatment must obviously depend on proper diagnosis, and *Common Symptoms of Disease in Children* is devoted to the diagnosis of children's ailments on the basis of their symptoms. With regard to infant feeding, behaviour problems and other conditions, I have referred to another book, *The Normal Child*. I have reduced my references to a few, in the hope that the family doctor who is not prepared to accept what I have written will look the matter up himself. I have also appended a separate list of books which may be usefully referred to for more detailed information.

I must express my thanks to the Editors of *Drug and Therapeutics Bulletin*, and of the *Prescribers' Journal*, because I have made so many quotations from their journals. Any good family doctor wishing to keep up to date should read these journals regularly; they are invaluable.

Finally, I wish to thank Mr. W.H. Toplis, Head Pharmacist at the Children's Hospital, for his invaluable help with details of dosage, preparations and costs; Dr. J.E. Struthers, of the Department of Health and Social Security, for some figures about prescribing rates; Dr. Hugh Halle, family doctor in Sheffield, for his most careful and valuable criticisms and suggestions after reading the script; Professor Donald Court, of Newcastle, for his customary kindness, thoroughness and honesty in criticism of the script; and my wife for all her help and comments. I have heeded all their criticisms, but the final version is my own, and may not always coincide with their views.

Finally, I wish to thank Miss Julia Grundy for typing the entire script, including the various drafts, so uncomplainingly.

Part 1
General Comments on Treatment

PRINCIPLES OF TREATMENT

I suggest that the following should be the principles underlying any treatment in children.

(A) Questions to ask before prescribing treatment

Before giving any treatment, one should ask oneself the following questions.

(1) *What good may it do?*
(2) *What harm may it do?*
(3) *What harm may be done by not giving the treatment?*

What good may it do? *In my opinion it is wrong to prescribe drugs which have no therapeutic value, on the grounds that the parents expect to be given a prescription.* In my experience in both general practice and in hospital a parent rarely expects a prescription when one has explained that no medicine will help, especially when one adds that medicine may be harmful, for all drugs have side effects. If the parents do insist, some placebo will have to be prescribed, but at least it must be both harmless and cheap. *No antibiotic should ever be prescribed as a placebo.* If the symptom is a cough, linctus simplex is all that is required.

IT IS HARMFUL, PSYCHOLOGICALLY UNSOUND AND EXPENSIVE TO PRESCRIBE DRUGS FOR NON-DISEASE OR FOR SIMPLE SELF-CURING CONDITIONS LIKE COLDS OR COMMON INFECTIOUS DISEASES WHICH ARE SELF-LIMITING AND WHICH CURE THEMSELVES AND ARE UNAFFECTED BY TREATMENT. When one considers the enormous sums of money paid by taxpayers for medicines, it is morally wrong to prescribe drugs costing millions of pounds when it is known that they have no pharmacological value and that many of them may do positive harm. THE PRESCRIBING OF DRUGS IS NO SUBSTITUTE FOR TALKING TO THE PARENTS. For instance, innumerable mothers in my Well Baby Clinic have complained that their young baby's nose gets blocked up. I have always told them that no nose drops are necessary, and that some Ear Nose and Throat specialists think that nose drops may damage the lining of the nose. Not a single mother after that has again asked me for a prescription for nose drops. It is wrong to prescribe a drug

3

for every symptom of which a patient complains, however trivial it is. There is no excuse for prescribing medicine for a baby's 'wind', or for a cold.

There is far too much unscientific nonsense in contemporary medical practice. A modern textbook recommends the following treatment for erythema nodosum: 'The child should be put on a light diet. Foci of infection should be looked for and, when found, cleared. Constipation should be corrected. Rest in bed should be insisted upon during the febrile period.' All four statements are nonsense. Erythema nodosum is usually a response to a streptococcal infection, though there are other causes, including drugs. There is no rationale whatsoever for any of the four lines of treatment recommended. None of them could possibly do the patient any good, and some of them, especially the removal of 'septic foci', which presumably include the tonsils, may do serious harm (see *Tonsillectomy*, p. 258).

It is not only wrong to prescribe drugs if they will achieve no good. It is wrong to demand restrictive measures, such as bed rest, limitation of exercise or diet, quarantine, isolation, confinement to the house or prevention from going to school; all do harm. Before any of these are prescribed there should be a good reason for them – a reason which can be defended before an intelligent parent or a scientific audience.

What harm may it do? All drugs have possible undesirable side effects, and many of these are dangerous. It follows that no drug should be prescribed unless (1) it is necessary to make the child better, (2) one is fully conversant with the possible side effects, and has balanced the need for the drug against the risk of giving it. Voltaire wrote that a physician is 'a person who pours drugs of which he knows little into a body of which he knows less'.

All operations carry a risk, particularly a risk from the anaesthetic. It has been calculated that cardiac arrest occurs in approximately 1 in every 2,300 anaesthetics given to children. Hence it is wrong to carry out or advise an operation on a child unless it is definitely in his interests. No operation should ever be performed on a child because the mother, father, aunt, mother-in-law or anyone else wants it to be done; the child alone matters. It is he who has to suffer the unpleasantness of the operation and its after effects or even complications. I have seen too many tragedies from totally unnecessary operations – including, for instance, a death under anaesthetic for a probing of the nasolachrymal duct which would have cured itself if only it had been left alone.

What harm may be done by not giving the treatment? In prescribing or arranging any potentially unpleasant or risky treatment or operation, one should ask oneself what harm would be done by not giving it. For instance, if a doctor wishes to remove the tonsils because of recurrent colds, he should ask all the three questions outlined above – What good will it do? (Answer: None): What harm may it do? (Answer: Plenty, including haemorrhage and death): What harm may be done by not doing it? (Answer: None). I would suggest that in this case it would be better not to do the operation.

(B) Follow-up

The child must be followed up so that one can be sure that the treatment has been effective, and so that one can learn from experience. *I feel that the commonest mistake in paediatric therapeutics is to fail to follow up in order to determine whether the diagnosis was correct and the treatment was successful.* For instance, it is inadequate to see a child once for acute otitis media, prescribe penicillin and not see him again to observe the response to treatment.

(C) The whole child

The whole child must be treated, and not just the presenting symptom. Doctors should aim at prevention as well as treatment, and when treating disease must always attend to the psychological factors, which may be much more important than the disease of which the child complains. Whatever the disease, any behaviour problems, whether apparently relevant to the illness or not, should be treated. It would be bad medical practice to treat a child for a cough and to fail to do anything about the obesity; to advise about the diet of a 9-month-old baby and to ignore the squint; to treat a child for abdominal pain and to fail to arrange for treatment of a lisp or of malocclusion or of malnutrition, just as it would be bad medical practice in the diagnostic field to examine a baby's chest and to fail to examine the hips for possible congenital subluxation, or to fail to make at least some estimate of the baby's developmental level.

(D) Talking to the parents and child

In a high proportion of cases seen by the family doctor or out-patient consultant, it is not medicine which is needed, but a discussion of the

problem with the parents. Certain commonly used expressions should never be used in a discussion with the parents, such as:
You are just being fussy.
You are just over-anxious.
There is nothing to be done.
He'll grow out of it.
It's just his nerves.
He's just lazy.
He wants a good hiding.

A good mother is 'fussy' and 'over-anxious', and nothing will infuriate her more than to be criticized for being 'over-anxious' about the child she loves. We have all seen innumerable examples of mothers being proved right when they insisted that there was something wrong with their child in spite of being told by a consultant or other doctor, 'There's nothing wrong with him. You're just being fussy.'

> A mother telephoned to me one evening to say that she was worried about her baby who was in my ward at the hospital, because she was sure that the problem was not just mismanagement of feeding, as she had been told. I promised to pick her up in my car in fifteen minutes at the telephone kiosk from which she had spoken to me, and to take her to the hospital where I would examine the child in her presence. There was a readily palpable pyloric tumour, and the necessary operation was performed later that evening.

> A mother took her month-old baby to a Casualty Department because she was sure that he was unwell. The Casualty Officer could find no abnormality, but the mother was so insistent that he asked a Registrar to see the baby. He too could find nothing, but the mother still maintained that the baby was not well. Almost against his will he performed a lumbar puncture and withdrew purulent cerebrospinal fluid.

It is easy to make the mistake of talking to the parents but failing to talk to the child. One of our greatest failures in paediatrics is failure to explain to the child as well as to the parents.

(E) The family

There are many circumstances in which it is not enough merely to treat the child. Almost all behaviour problems in the child are treated not by prescribing medicines for the child, and not by giving him formal psycho-therapy, but by attention to the environment, especially the management of the child at home and school, and by guiding the parents in their attitude to him. In particular they need to know about the child's need for love and security, wise discipline and acceptance, and for the gradual acquisition of independence.

There are circumstances in which the treatment of the child consists not in giving him medicine, but in treating his mother's anaemia, which she did not know was the cause of her fatigue, bad temper and intolerance, or his mother's thyrotoxicosis, which she did not know was the cause of her psychological symptoms which were reflected in the behaviour of her child.

Skin or antrum infections in the child may have to be treated not only by attention to the child's symptoms, but by attention to the reservoir of infection in another member of the family, or to the lack of cleanliness in the family.

It is a common failing to overtreat the child and undertreat the rest of the family.

(F) The good doctor must know when he does not know

No doctor, whether consultant or general practitioner, is good at every-thing. Every doctor must know the limits of his knowledge, and know when to seek help from someone else – a consultant or other person more experienced in the problem in question.

(G) Polypharmacy: Drug combinations

Drug combinations are widely advocated by drug firms, but rarely recom-mended by clinicians or by textbooks. *It is far wiser to prescribe drugs singly in the dosage required than in combination, for drugs may interact with each other and interfere with the treatment. When side effects occur, one does not know which drug has caused them; and drug combinations are nearly always more expensive than single drugs.* In the words of an article in *Drug and Therapeutics Bulletin* (1967), 'the effects of any single drug are seldom confined to the effect desired by the prescriber. It is becoming clearer that the simultaneous use of two or more potent drugs makes a complicated matter more complicated. It is therefore best not to use combined therapy, or preparations containing more than one drug, un-less there is a clear advantage to the patient.'

References

ANON. (1967) Drug interactions. *Drug and Therapeutics Bulletin*, 5, 89.
BERGMANN A.B. & STAMM S.J. (1967) The morbidity of cardiac non disease in school children. *New England J. Med.* 276, 1008.

THE SICK CHILD

The attitude to illness. *A person's whole attitude to illness is likely to be implanted in the early years of life.* The family doctor has an important responsibility to guide the parents in this. If they show great anxiety and make a fuss about every trivial symptom or about every abrasion to the knee, the child must be expected to respond more and more to every trivial injury and symptom and to magnify it. The child's attitude begins as a conscious desire for attention, but soon it becomes subconscious and he really 'feels' the imaginary symptom or exaggerates it in his mind. In a Casualty Department it is interesting to observe the different responses of children who have suffered a minor injury; some are violently hysterical, while others are entirely calm and stoical. The difference lies partly in the child's personality, but largely in the attitude which the parents have displayed in the past. When a child is put to bed for every trivial symptom, every complaint of abdominal discomfort, diarrhoea, cold or headache, and given medicines, petted and fussed, and the family doctor is brought in, the parents are asking him to become an adult neurotic and a hypochondriac. When they keep him off school for every trivial symptom and keep him indoors because he has a cold, they are implanting in him a wrong idea of the importance of his symptoms – and incidentally giving him a wrong idea of the importance of education and encouraging him to be lazy.

Parents must strike the delicate balance between sympathy and insensitivity. When the child falls, they should see that he has not broken his leg, but otherwise they should ignore the injury until he gets home, when the graze may be cleansed. Every effort should be made to encourage a child not to exaggerate his symptoms – one of the bases of adult neurosis.

Parents should themselves set a good example with regard to their own illnesses and symptoms; it is inevitable that the child will imitate them. If the parents are constantly complaining about headache, indigestion, wind, fatigue or other symptoms, and miss no opportunity to discuss these symptoms and their fears of illness in front of the children, they must expect their children to develop symptoms – either in direct imitation, or as attention-seeking devices, or in subconscious fear that they will suffer as their parents do.

There may well be a relation between absenteeism in adult life and childhood attitudes to illness, instilled by the parents through their overt expressions of anxiety, and by the father's own behaviour with regard to illness and absence from work. If a father absents himself from work for any trivial symptom (or worse still, for no symptoms at all), it will not be surprising if the child adopts a similar attitude to school and later to his job. The family doctor can do much to guide parents in these attitudes.

Food and fluid. When a child is feverish, he loses his appetite. Children have a compensatory increase of appetite following an infection, and the parents need to be reassured that the children will not suffer an eventual reduction in weight as a result of the illness. They should not try to make them eat.

It is essential to try to persuade young children to drink extra fluid during a febrile illness. Every children's ward or hospital is used to admitting babies or small children with severe acidosis and uraemia as a result of insufficient fluid intake in simple respiratory infections. Children with acute asthma may become considerably dehydrated for the same reason.

General management. Parents have to relax discipline when a child is ill. It is useless to attempt to teach discipline to a child feeling poorly. Discipline should be reimposed as soon as he is better.

If the child has been allowed to sleep in the parents' room when he is ill, he should be returned to his own room immediately he has passed the acute stage. Many bad habits begin with an illness.

Every effort should be made to keep the child occupied when he is poorly. This is much easier if proper advice is taken as to keeping him in bed. The child should be kept in bed only if he feels unfit to get up, and if there is a good scientific reason for keeping him there.

It is important to avoid suggesting symptoms. A few minutes after I had told a mother in my ward that I had found no evidence of organic disease in her boy who complained of recurrent abdominal pains, she was overheard saying to him, 'Of course you have tummy ache, darling, haven't you?' He had.

Parents should understand that when a child has recently acquired sphincter control, he is apt to have an accident and wet the bed when poorly, or to soil his pants when he has diarrhoea. A child may be very upset when this happens, and he needs comforting.

REFERRAL TO HOSPITAL ADVISED

I once carried out a survey of 100 consecutive deaths of infants in the home under 1 year of age, in order to determine how many had been seen by a paediatrician in the home or in hospital for his illness. Only four had been seen by a specialist or hospital doctor.

In this section I have excluded conditions which one can be certain would always be referred to a hospital (*e.g.* exomphalos, severe head injury with fracture of the skull, etc.).

Below are some important examples of conditions for which the child should be sent to hospital – if only for a specialist opinion, but usually for specialist treatment.

VOMITING. Newborn vomiting bile-stained or green material (intestinal obstruction until proved otherwise).

Newborn vomiting and ill. (May be meningitis, intestinal obstruction, uraemia, etc.)

Baby of about 4–6 weeks with projectile vomiting, one big vomit immediately after or during a feed. Suggests congenital pyloric stenosis, rapidly curable by operation. It is a mistake to attempt to treat it by atropine methylnitrate.

Vomiting, for which no cause has been found, persisting for over 12 hours. It may be due to intestinal obstruction or other serious cause.

Vomiting with abdominal distension (possible intestinal obstruction or perforation of a viscus).

Vomiting baby, with blood in vomit. May be hiatus hernia.

DIARRHOEA (Gastroenteritis) in a baby or toddler, unless child is well. In view of the rapid yet insidious development of severe dehydration, any infant with diarrhoea and vomiting who is treated at home will have to be seen at least twice a day until he is obviously improving, so that any deterioration can lead to immediate referral to hospital.

MELAENA OR HAEMATEMESIS, neonatal. Blood loss may demand an urgent transfusion.

JAUNDICE on the first day. This is haemolytic disease until proved otherwise. Treatment is urgent to prevent serious brain damage.

Jaundice in newborn baby, at first thought to be physiological, but not clearing (*e.g.* within a week). It may be septicaemia. Prolonged physiological jaundice may be related to cretinism.

NEWBORN BABY CHOKING ON FEED, or with apparent inability to swallow saliva. May be oesophageal atresia.

CYANOSIS AND CHOKING IN NEWBORN BABY, relieved as soon as he cries. May be choanal atresia.

CYANOTIC ATTACKS or persistent cyanosis in newborn baby.

LARYNGEAL STRIDOR, acute (*e.g.* due to acute laryngotracheobronchitis). Complete obstruction may develop with alarming rapidity and fatal results.

INCREASING RESPIRATION RATE IN NEWBORN BABY. May be respiratory distress syndrome or other serious condition (*e.g.* diaphragmatic hernia).

PNEUMONIA IN A BABY. Apart from the inherent danger of pneumonia in an infant, the possibility of an error in diagnosis must be remembered. It may be heart failure (*e.g.* congenital heart disease or paroxysmal tachycardia).

SUDDEN OR SEVERE UNEXPLAINED COUGH. The possibility of a foreign body should be remembered.

SEVERE ATTACK OF ASTHMA, not responding to the usual home treatment. Status asthmaticus is a serious emergency and may be fatal.

A PURULENT NASAL DISCHARGE not improving after a fortnight.

A DISCHARGING EAR.

SUSPECTED DEAFNESS at any age, and delayed speech.

SQUINT IN A BABY after six months. Neglect may cause blindness in the squinting eye. A retinoblastoma may present in early infancy as a squint.

CONVULSIONS – p. 126.

UNEXPLAINED DROWSINESS. May be meningitis.

NECK STIFFNESS. This must never be assumed to be due to an infection such as otitis media or pneumonia; the child may have meningitis.

HEADACHE developing as a new symptom in a previously well child.

URINARY TRACT INFECTION. It is far better to establish the diagnosis in hospital, where the necessary facilities are available, where there are personnel trained in obtaining a clean specimen, where the causative organism with its sensitivity can be determined, and where the necessary radiological examination can be performed, than to guess at the diagnosis in the home, guessing the correct treatment and guessing that the cure is complete. The result of a faulty guess may be chronic pyelonephritis, hypertension and death in later childhood or early adult life.

ABDOMINAL PAIN acute, any age. Rhythmical attacks of abdominal pain with pallor and perhaps vomiting in an infant or young child (possible intussusception).

INGUINAL HERNIA. It is wrong to wait until it strangulates.

INFLAMMATION over bone; it may be due to osteitis.

AN UNEXPLAINED LIMP.

RHEUMATIC FEVER.

POISONING OF ANY KIND. The worst mistake is to be misled by the dangerous latent asymptomatic period, especially in the case of iron, diphenoxylate (lomotil) or salicylate poisoning.

Transport to hospital

The family doctor has some responsibility with regard to the way in which a sick child is taken to hospital. For instance, he should see that the infant is kept warm. This may sound obvious, but there must be few paediatricians who have not seen infants arrive at hospital with a subnormal temperature suffering from the dangerous and often fatal 'cold injury'. The ambulance may be equipped with an incubator heated by the vehicle itself or by its own battery or other heating system; but it is wise to check this before the baby is removed to the hospital. It is also important that the child should not be overheated.

When a child has ingested poison, he is transported in the prone ('spank') position, so as to reduce the risk of inhaling vomit.

BED

'Teach us to live that we may dread
Unnecessary time in bed.
Get people up and we may save
Our patients from an early grave.'

(Asher 1947)

Sir Melville Arnott wrote in 1954: 'It is widely regarded as normal for the sick person to be in bed. The attitude is such that the burden of proof is on the physician who says the patient should not be in bed rather than the reverse, which I believe is the only logical position. Once that is accepted, then it becomes illogical to allow or encourage confinement to bed without good and sufficient evidence of its beneficial effect. In most hospitals, even today, the patient is expected to be in bed; the whole organization is geared to such a state, and there is little provision for the up-patient.'

I agree entirely with what Browse wrote (1965) in his excellent monograph on the physiological and pathological consequences of bed rest: 'The bed is often a sign of our therapeutic inadequacy, rather than a therapeutic measure deserving of praise. The bed is *the* non-specific treatment of our time, *the* great placebo.'

Parents and others have a touching faith in the magic power of the bed to cure almost anything; but they do not stop to think how it is supposed to achieve the cure.

I am convinced that far too many children are kept in bed quite unnecessarily. I have visited hospitals in many countries, including Russia, Scandinavia, Egypt, Palestine, Yugoslavia, Italy, Switzerland, France, Austria, Australia and the United States, and in almost all these hospitals I have seen children kept in bed for no reason which I was able to discern. In one European capital I saw an entire ward full of children with behaviour problems; they were admitted, put to bed and kept there for a month or so until the time came for their discharge. In another city on the Continent I saw a ward full of children with epilepsy – all in bed. In both these cities I could not discover why the children had been admitted at all.

Some years ago, when my ward was full, I admitted a well girl for investigation of albuminuria. In the afternoon on my ward round I found

13

her in bed, and asked why she was not up and about. The ward sister said, 'Because no one gave me instructions to that effect.' I replied that the reasonable thing was to have the patient up and about unless someone gave instructions that she should stay in bed. I could not think why it should be thought that recovery from any disease she had, if there was disease, would be made more rapid by keeping her in bed for the day or two during which our investigations were being carried out.

When a child is admitted to hospital it is assumed by many that he will be put to bed, whatever the condition for which he is admitted. I have never understood the rationale of bed rest for most medical conditions. I believe that the commonest reason for keeping a child in bed in hospital is simply that no one has thought of getting him up.

In the home the same irrational treatment is apt to be ordered. If a child with chickenpox, mumps, rubella, whooping cough, a cold, tonsillitis, bronchitis, asthma, diarrhoea, abdominal discomfort, a headache or a raised temperature wants to sit in a chair or on the floor, reading or playing a game, I can see no reason why he should not do so. No one has yet been able to explain why a child should recover more quickly sitting up in bed than sitting up in a chair. Will contact between the child's buttocks and the bed lead to a more rapid recovery than contact between his buttocks and a chair? It seems most unlikely to me that a child with chickenpox or German measles will lose his spots more quickly, become non-infectious sooner, or recover more rapidly if he is kept in bed.

Is it thought that a child has more rest on a bed than on a chair? That is quite untrue. It has been proved that a child in bed is more active than a child out of bed; in any case I cannot see why rest should be necessary for a child with chickenpox or any of the other conditions mentioned. It would be much more sensible to let the child regulate his own activity according to how he feels.

Unnecessary confinement to bed makes sleep at night more difficult; it bores the child, partly because it is less easy for him to play games or read; and it tends to isolate him from his siblings. If prolonged, it predisposes to obesity, and may lead to a variety of metabolic changes, including decreased nitrogen retention and increased loss of calcium and phosphorus. The danger of renal calculus formation in children immobilized for orthopaedic conditions is well known.

An American family doctor (Gibson 1956) carried out a controlled study of bed rest in 1,082 children with acute respiratory infections. He divided them into two groups: one group had to remain in bed for at least three days, and the other group were allowed to be up and about if they wished. The groups were comparable as to sex, colour, age, illness and medicines given. There was no difference between the groups in the duration of either fever or illness. He wrote, 'As time went by, a distinct impression began to form that the children with a high temperature who were up and about seemed to get well just as quickly as the better-controlled children who stayed in bed.'

In the appropriate sections I have discussed the role of bed rest in rheumatic fever, rheumatoid arthritis, acute nephritis, the nephrotic syndrome and tuberculosis, and I express the view that if the patient is well enough to be up and about, it is better that he should be. In the section on poliomyelitis I have mentioned the desirability of bed rest in the pre-paralytic febrile stage, and in the section on infective hepatitis the doubts about bed rest as compared with reasonable activity. In the section on muscular dystrophy I have emphasized the positive harm done by keeping a child in bed.

References

ARNOTT W.M. (1954) The abuse of rest. *Lancet*, 1, 1251.

ASHER R.A.J. (1947) The dangers of going to bed. *Brit. Med. J.* 2, 967.

BASS H.N. & SCHULMAN J.L. (1967) Quantitative assessment of children's activity in and out of bed. *Am. J. Dis. Child.* 113, 242.

BERGMAN A.B. & STAMM S.J. (1967) The morbidity of cardiac non-disease in school children. *New England J. Med.* 276, 1008.

BROWSE N.L. (1965) *The Physiology and Pathology of Bed Rest.* Springfield, Charles Thomas.

GIBSON J.P. (1956) How much bed rest is necessary for children with fever? *J. Pediat.* 49, 256.

ILLINGWORTH R.S. (1963) Why put him to bed? *Clinical Pediatrics*, 2, 108.

DIET

There is a great deal of unscientific nonsense about special diets. There are, of course, various metabolic diseases for which a special diet is necessary. These include abnormal aminoacidurias, in particular phenyl-ketonuria, but including tyrosinosis, leucinosis, histidinaemia, hyper-glycinaemia; hypercalcaemia, carbohydrate intolerance, galactosaemia, coeliac disease, nephrogenic diabetes insipidus, leucine sensitivity, abeta-lipoproteinaemia, and hyperlipidaemia. An occasional child is allergic to certain foodstuffs, such as eggs or milk protein, which must therefore be avoided. Some migraine sufferers are upset by foods containing tyramine, such as chocolate and cheese. A high protein diet may be reasonably pre-scribed for children with fibrocystic disease of the pancreas. The obese child should avoid sweets, cut down fried food and reduce carbohydrate intake.

But there are many other conditions for which special diets are still prescribed unnecessarily. Textbooks tend to advise a 'light diet' for a variety of conditions, which in fact do not call for any alteration in diet. In febrile conditions the child should be allowed to adjust his own diet to what he can take. In acute nephritis, there is no need to restrict protein unless there is severe oliguria, and there is certainly no case for protein restriction after the acute stage, whether there is residual albuminuria or not. A high protein diet in the nephrotic syndrome achieves little, while in cirrhosis of the liver it can do more harm than good. The common prescription for diabetes mellitus is now a free diet without excesses.

In diseases of the alimentary tract, diets are of little value. Salter (1969) wrote: 'In most of these gastroenterological disorders for which diets are regarded as an important aspect of therapy, there is little evidence to show that their use achieves anything other than the relief of symptoms, and even this may occasionally be open to doubt. In consequence, the patient should be deprived of the pleasure of a normal diet only when there is good evidence of likely benefit. Most special diets are unpleasant, expen-sive, difficult to adhere to, tedious to prepare, and cause considerable inconvenience.' Palmer (1967) wrote that 'diet is no more than a gesture' in gastrointestinal disorders. A roughage-free diet is unnecessary in ulcerative colitis, but an occasional patient seems to fare better on a milk-free diet.

When an infant has gastroenteritis it is customary to stop the intake of all food (but not fluid) for 24 hours, and this treatment is widely accep-ted.

For the treatment of infective hepatitis a fat-free diet should not be prescribed: the patient should himself decide how much fat he can take.

In the treatment of epilepsy which is refractory to all the normal drug therapy a ketogenic diet may be used, but it is expensive and disliked by the patients.

It used to be the practice to restrict all fat in children with so-called acidosis attacks, which are now known to be related to migraine; it was not realized that the ketosis was the result, not the cause, of the attacks. *Children should not be put on to a special diet unless there is sound scientific justification for it. Unnecessary dieting leads to food fads and dietary invalidism. It is unfair and unkind to a child to put him on to an entirely unnecessary restrictive diet.*

References

FRANCIS D.E.M. & DIXON D.J.W. (1969) *Diets for Sick Children.* Oxford, Blackwell Scientific Publications.

PALMER E.D. (1967) *Functional Gastrointestinal Disorders.* Baltimore, Williams & Wilkins.

SALTER R.H. (1969) What should the patient eat? *Lancet,* 1, 869.

ON KEEPING THE CHILD OFF SCHOOL

In my opinion far too many children are quite unnecessarily kept off school. Mothers feel lonely when all the children are at school, and welcome any excuse to have a child at home. Education suffers, and children should not be kept at home without a good reason. In the section on asthma I have drawn attention to the vicious circle which is set up by keeping the child at home for every wheeze; he drops behind in his work, worries about it and wheezes all the more. There is no point in keeping the child at home because he has a cold or a cough following a cold. It is not clear why it should be thought that a child with a cough will get better more quickly if he goes shopping with his mother, goes to the cinema and visits the welfare clinic with his baby sister, rather than if he goes to school. Children are kept away far too long for the common infectious diseases. After each section on these diseases I have added the duration of infectivity. For instance, a child is infectious with rubella for two or three days after the development of the rash, and with chickenpox for a week after the rash has developed. Yet children are commonly kept off school for two weeks for rubella and three weeks for chickenpox.

Bransby (1951) showed that at any one time in a British city 10 per cent of children are away from school, and that absences are much more frequent in the lower social classes, large families, children with a low IQ,

B

children in the lower streams at school, and children from poor class districts. Under the age of 7, 12 per cent of absences were for non-medical reasons; from 8 to 11 years, 20 per cent; over 12 years, 30 per cent. A child with a normal temperature should be kept off school only if there is a good scientific reason. Unnecessary absences from school have a bad effect on the child's education, implant in him a wrong attitude to work, and encourage laziness and exaggeration of the importance of his symptoms.

References

BRANSBY E.R. (1951) A study of absence from school. *Medical Officer*, 86, 223, 237.
SMITH R.E. (1947) Incubation and isolation at school. *Lancet*, 2, 1.
SMITH R.E. (1963) Quarantine. *Brit. Med. J.* 2, 374.

COMMON MISTAKES IN TREATMENT

I hope that no one will think that in writing this section I am criticizing doctors. I want simply to draw attention to the common and important mistakes made by doctors working with children in hospital or at home.

(1) *Convulsions.* It is a common mistake to ascribe convulsions to teething, to confuse grand mal with petit mal, and to confuse febrile convulsions with epilepsy. Infantile spasms are commonly overlooked or confused with petit mal. (For the differential diagnosis, see p. 126.)

The commonest mistake in the treatment of grand mal is inadequacy of treatment (see p. 160).

(2) *Pyogenic meningitis.* It is a disaster to miss the diagnosis of pyogenic meningitis in the home, for delayed or wrong treatment may involve serious sequelae or death. Yet it does not often occur in the experience of any family doctor; its possibility has to be remembered in any febrile illness. It is wrong to prescribe antibiotics for a child with meningism, or for a child with drowsiness and vomiting or a suspected febrile convulsion, for if the child has meningitis, antibiotics make it difficult or impossible for the hospital doctor to culture the organism and therefore to prescribe the appropriate treatment. The common absence of bulging of the

fontanelle or of meningism in the baby or toddler leads to errors in diagnosis.

(3) *Otitis media.* Failure to make the diagnosis may lead to rupture of the drum, and failure to prescribe proper antibiotic treatment may lead to chronic thickening of the drum and deafness. The treatment of otitis media emphatically does not consist of 'drops' – except perhaps occasionally analgesic drops – and these are unnecessary and may cause harm by sensitization.

(4) *Teething. Teething does not cause convulsions, diarrhoea, fever, bronchitis or a rash.* Treatment of convulsions or fever as teething may and frequently does lead to a tragedy.

(5) *Acute laryngeal stridor and laryngotracheobronchitis.* Failure to recognize the rapidity with which a stridor can progress, so that complete obstruction occurs, is a serious mistake which may lead to death. If the child is not referred to hospital, frequent visits (*e.g.* two or three times a day) are necessary until improvement commences.

(6) *Gastroenteritis.* Failure to recognize the rapidity with which serious dehydration occurs may lead to death or residual cerebral damage. A baby with gastroenteritis can never be treated 'on the telephone'. If the child is not referred to hospital, frequent visits are needed (*e.g.* two or three a day) until improvement commences. Dehydration in an overweight baby is particularly easy to miss.

(7) *Foreign body in the bronchus.* Many disasters occur as a result of prescribing cough medicine for a child who has a peanut or other foreign body in the bronchus. The diagnosis may be suspected on a history of a sudden onset of a cough, stridor or wheeze, without an obvious respiratory infection, but there is not always this story. Failure of a cough to clear should lead the family doctor to refer the child to hospital for diagnosis.

(8) *Asthma.* Failure to recognize the seriousness of status asthmaticus and therefore failure to refer him to hospital for urgent admission may lead to the child's death.

(9) *Poisons.* Failure to recognize the latent period after ingestion of iron, salicylates or other poisons may lead to serious illness. Every case of poisoning should be referred to hospital.

(10) *Maltreatment* of surgical conditions due to errors in diagnosis, in particular congenital pyloric stenosis, appendicitis, intussusception, intestinal obstruction, strangulated hernia.

(11) *Diabetes.* Wrong treatment due to failure to examine the urine.

(12) *Haemolytic disease of the newborn.* Failure to arrange for Rhesus negative mothers with antibodies to be delivered in hospital. Failure to

refer the baby to hospital when jaundice develops on the first day – because of failure to remember that jaundice on the first day must be regarded as due to haemolytic disease until proved otherwise.

(13) *Administration* of iron for suspected but non-proven anaemia.

(14) *Wrong management* of crying by the infant or toddler at night, on the grounds that it is due to wind or indigestion – always a wrong diagnosis – rather than mismanagement by the parents.

(15) *In the case of the breast-fed baby*, ascribing infrequent stools (which are normal) to constipation, and therefore giving laxatives, or ascribing frequent stools (which are normal) to diarrhoea. It is common to ascribe symptoms to the breast milk 'not suiting the baby' – a diagnosis which is always wrong except in very rare metabolic diseases.

A common mistake is to ascribe symptoms, such as crying, to over-feeding. Overfeeding in a young breast-fed baby is a myth.

(16) *In the artificially fed baby*, ascribing symptoms to the dried milk 'not suiting the baby' – a diagnosis which is always wrong except in the rare metabolic diseases. Except in these, it is never necessary to change from one dried milk to another in order to find one which suits the baby.

Mistakes based on pharmacological errors

(1) *Antibiotics.* Probably the commonest mistake based on errors in pharmacological knowledge is the abuse of antibiotics – the prescription of antibiotics for virus conditions such as colds, or for non-infective conditions such as asthma, or for the treatment of bacterial infections to which they are known to be insensitive. It is a dangerous mistake to prescribe chloramphenicol for respiratory infections, such as bronchitis or laryngitis, because of the risk of damage to the bone marrow. It is wrong to prescribe antibiotics for a child merely to reassure the mother when one knows that there is no pharmacological indication for them. They are expensive, may have side effects, and may lead to drug resistance which will in future involve the use of still more costly drugs which may be less effective.

(2) *Diarrhoea.* Treatment of mild diarrhoea by kaolin, which from its nature could hardly be expected to have a pharmacological action when dispersed through many feet of intestine, or worse still by antibiotics. The great majority of cases of diarrhoea are self-limiting, and in the case of mild salmonella or shigella dysentery infections, antibiotics not only do no good, but may do harm (see *Diarrhoea*, p. 145).

(3) *The prescription of potassium citrate* for urinary tract infections, instead of the establishment of a precise diagnosis followed by the appropriate antibiotic.

(4) *Cough medicines.* It is highly doubtful whether any so-called 'expectorant' cough medicine loosens the sputum, except potassium iodide (which may produce a goitre). Cough suppressants are rarely advisable in children and usually contraindicated. A vast amount of money is spent on useless cough medicines for a self-limiting condition, such as influenza, requiring no treatment.

(5) *Phenobarbitone and tranquillizers.* Phenobarbitone is virtually never of value in the treatment of behaviour problems in children. Given for over-activity, it may have the paradoxical effect of making the behaviour worse.

Tranquillizing drugs are rarely needed for children, and virtually never for normal children.

Phenobarbitone and tranquillizing drugs tend to be used as a substitute, and a most ineffective substitute, for talking to the parents about the management of the child.

(6) *Tonics and vitamins.* There is no such thing as a tonic; it is futile to prescribe a so-called 'tonic'.

There is no place for additional vitamins after infancy for a child receiving a normal diet.

There are still people who give their children codliver oil and malt or similar preparations for no apparent reason.

(7) *Failure to be aware of side effects of drugs.* No one can remember all the possible side effects of drugs. I have included a fairly comprehensive list on p. 30.

Other mistakes

It is unnecessary to use expensive drugs when there are equivalent non-proprietary preparations which are much cheaper.

Restrictive practices. These include keeping a child indoors, in bed, off school, on a special diet, restricting physical education at school, or limiting exercise in children with congenital heart disease or children who have had rheumatic fever. All these are discussed in the appropriate sections.

Treating non-disease or self-limiting disease, when no treatment is necessary, and where the treatment will not help the child. Many prescribe nose drops for babies when they have a cold; they are totally unnecessary and may damage the mucosa. There is rarely need to prescribe medicine for an elevated temperature; this is best dealt with by removal of excess clothing and by tepid sponging. There is no need to prescribe medicine for colds or influenza.

Lack of knowledge of the normal. This applies particularly to surgical treatment for gum cysts in babies, tongue tie, the alveolar frenum, probing of the nasolachrymal duct, strawberry naevi, tonsils, undescended but in fact retractile testes.

Failure to treat the whole child. Treating a child for a presenting symptom, but failing to treat or arrange treatment for a squint, lisp, stutter, malocclusion, dental caries or obesity.

Overconfidence or failure to follow up to ensure that the treatment has been successful and that the diagnosis was correct.

Failure to treat the rest of the family, where relevant. This applies particularly to scabies, but also to pyogenic infections, including chronic antrum suppuration, in which the trouble is kept going by a reservoir of infection in another member of the family.

Treatment on the telephone. It is rarely safe to give advice about a sick child on the telephone without going to see him. It is unlikely that there is any paediatrician who has not seen tragic consequences from this practice – particularly in the case of abdominal pain, gastroenteritis or stridor.

A diagnostic snare. When there is an epidemic of some infection such as influenza, it is particularly easy to assume that, when a child's symptoms resemble those of numerous other patients suffering from the prevalent infection, these symptoms are due to that infection. For instance, when a doctor has seen ten consecutive patients with influenza, and then sees a child with cough, fever and headache, he assumes that the child has influenza too – while in fact he has pyogenic meningitis, or an inhaled foreign body.

When a child has recurrent attacks of a condition such as migraine, and advice is sought about the child having another attack with similar symptoms, it is easy to conclude that the child merely has another attack of migraine, when in fact he is suffering from acute appendicitis or meningitis.

TRADE NAMES AND OFFICIAL NAMES

Some official names are difficult to memorize, but the multitude of trade names for some preparations is thoroughly confusing and may lead to danger. Throughout this book I have used the official names, but have always included the principal trade names so as to reduce confusion.

I was asked to see a boy who was suffering from asthma; he was being given ten different drugs, of which three contained isoprenaline – a fact concealed under trade names. He was lucky to survive. I was asked to see a boy suffering from epilepsy, and prescribed phenytoin and primidone. When I saw him a month later his mother said, 'Shall I continue to give him the Epanutin and Mysoline?' I had neglected to ask whether he was already receiving the drugs from a previous doctor. All four bottles were properly labelled, but the mother did not know that Epanutin is phenytoin and that Mysoline is primidone. The boy suffered no side effects from the double dosage. The confusion caused by the large number of trade names for some drugs can well be imagined by glancing at p. 23, where some of the trade names for the tetracyclines are listed, and p. 65, where trade names for penicillin are supplied.

Besides the importance of avoiding confusion, there is a further reason for using official names rather than trade names – cost. It may be significantly cheaper to prescribe a drug under its official name than under a trade name, though the drugs are identical. If doctors in this country prescribed just five drugs under their official names – chlorpheniramine, nitrofurantoin, imipramine, phenytoin, and paracetamol – almost £1,400,000 would be saved each year.

DRUGS, DOSAGE AND ADMINISTRATION

I know of no short cut for calculating the dose of a drug for a child. Various methods have been advocated, such as calculation of the dose by surface area or weight, or by allowing a percentage of the adult dose for certain age periods of childhood. All the methods have advantages and disadvantages. The family doctor cannot be expected to work out a child's surface area and he may not know the weight. Furthermore, if the child is fat, the weight would not give a good indication of the dose, because fat plays little part in drug metabolism. Calculation of the dose by weight (*e.g.* of a sulphonamide) may be satisfactory in early childhood but may lead to serious overdosage in an older child. Some drugs (*e.g.* chloramphenicol) are particularly dangerous in the newborn period, and the dose cannot be worked out on the basis of a percentage of the adult dose. Babies and children are much more tolerant of certain drugs (*e.g.* phenobarbitone) than are adults, so that a much bigger dose has to be given than one would expect from adult requirements. A dehydrated baby, or a child with liver or kidney disease, needs less than the usual dose. The dose cannot be accurately measured on the basis of weight if there is oedema. There are many variables which make any one method of calculating the dose for a child unsatisfactory. It is better for the doctor to know the dose of a few frequently used drugs and have a ready source of reference (*e.g.* the National Formulary) for the others.

For many purposes, Catzel's method is reasonable; he suggested that as an approximate guide one should reckon the dose as follows:

Child's age	*Percentage of dose for 65 kg. adult*
12 years	75
7 years	50
1 year	25
Newborn	12·5

For a fat child, one calculates the dose on the basis of three-quarters of the normal dose; for a dehydrated child the dose will be less than that of a normal child. In this book I have supplied the dose, and named the available preparations after each section if they are not given in the script.

Few children under the age of 5 are able to take a tablet or capsule – or at least a large tablet. A tablet can often be crushed (between two spoons, if necessary) and given with jam, honey or apple, and may be much preferred to a flavoured suspension or syrup. Tablets are much cheaper than suspensions, syrups or other liquid preparations. A liquid should be measured by the 5 ml. plastic teaspoon supplied – because ordinary teaspoons and tablespoons vary considerably in size; for quantities over 5 ml. a measuring glass should be used.

It is most undesirable to have a fight with a child about taking a medicine. If a fight occurs once, it is likely to occur again; some of the dose may be lost and some may find its way into the trachea. Medicine should never be given in a baby's feeding bottle – partly because some of it may be left.

No intramuscular injection should ever be given into the arm; the danger of a nerve palsy is far too great. The safest place for an intramuscular injection is the outer side of the middle of the thigh, pointing the needle in a horizontal direction at right angles to the femur and to the long axis of the leg.

In the case of penicillin, there is much to be said for giving the first dose intramuscularly if the child is ill. If one uses a mixed long and short acting preparation such as 'Triplopen', one knows that there will be a good blood level for 24–48 hours; after 24 hours one continues the treatment by mouth.

The danger of addiction must always be remembered. It would be wrong to introduce an older child to amphetamine, phenmetrazine or other drugs of addiction (*e.g.* for the treatment of obesity).

References

Anon. (1963) Dosage. *Drug and Therapeutics Bulletin*, 1, 69.
Catzel P. (1966) *Paediatric Prescriber*, 3rd ed. Oxford, Blackwell Scientific Publications.
Leach R.H. & Wood B.S.B. (1967) Drug dosage for children. *Lancet*, 2, 1350.
Wade O.L. & McDevitt G.D. (1966) Prescribing and the British National Formulary. *Brit. Med. J.* 2, 635.

SAFETY WITH DRUGS AND POISONS

Many thousands of children are admitted every year to British hospitals with poisoning. The commonest poisons taken by children are salicylates, barbiturates, ferrous sulphate, laxatives, heart pills, cosmetics, plants and berries, pesticides, paints and contraceptive pills. The family doctor can make an important contribution to the problem. The following instructions to the parent are important:

1 Never leave medicine at the child's bedside.

2 Except only in the case of an older school child with a reliable personality, never leave the child with a supply of tablets or other medicine with which to treat himself.

3 Discard all unused medicine prescribed for the child or other members of the family; do not throw it away to a place where children can get it.

4 Never put medicine into a lemonade or similar bottle.

5 Do not refer to medicine as 'sweets'.

6 Put all drugs and poisons out of reach of the child. Poisons should be in a poison cupboard and the key should be removed.

7 Never let a child see you hide a drug or poison. It is a challenge to him to get it.

8 It is better not to allow a small child to see one taking medicine or giving it to another child. The older one may imitate, take it himself, or give it to a sibling.

9 Never store medicines or poisons on a food shelf.

10 Never give medicine without first reading the label on the bottle. Never give it in the dark.

11 The nature and name of the tablets or medicine should be clearly written on the bottle – in accordance with the recommendations of the British Pharmaceutical Society, the British Medical Association, the National Formulary Committee and others.

12 Do not give the child aspirins flavoured as sweets.

ABUSE OF DRUGS

Few doctors can doubt that there is overprescribing in home and hospital, and that far too many drugs are being taken. In England and Wales in 1968, 271 million prescriptions were dispensed, at a cost of £146m. There were 20 million prescriptions for hypnotics, 12 million for tranquillizers and 4½ million for pep pills. It is said that every year the British Public consumes 30,000 gallons of liquid paraffin, has 3½ million prescriptions for laxatives, and spends an addition £5m. on laxatives from chemists' shops. In this country there are 15 million prescriptions for penicillin in one year. In the same year in the United States one billion prescriptions were dispensed, twice as many as ten years ago – the equivalent of five prescriptions for every man, woman and child. In 1968, over 5 million prescriptions for liquid preparations of penicillin were written in England and Wales, providing enough for 25 teaspoonsful for every pre-school child in the country. In addition, twice as many non-prescribed medicines were taken. In the Johns Hopkins Hospital, Baltimore (*International Medical Digest* 1967), the average number of drugs prescribed per patient on the medical service was 10–12, and some patients received as many as 50 drugs. Some years ago it was said that Americans spent $830m. on quack medicines – more than the entire cost of health education and medical research in America. Every day, 21 tons of aspirins are used in the United States.

Some years ago Bryant (1955) found that only 8 of 503 infants under a year of age studied by him had not been given unprescribed drugs, and Creery in the same year found that 93 per cent of 200 normal infants had been given alkalis, 79 per cent magnesia, and 66 per cent carminatives. It need hardly be said that in no case would alkalis or carminatives be justifiable. There is never any need to give a carminative to a baby or child of any age. It is rarely necessary to prescribe magnesia for an infant; constipation, if present at all, is better corrected by adjusting the fluid and fruit intake.

Perhaps the worst abuse of all is that of the antibiotic. It is little short of a tragedy that such vast sums are spent on antibiotics for cases in which there is no indication at all of their need. One constantly sees children who have been given, for every cold, sniffle, cough or wheeze, antibiotics which could not possibly do any good. In one year in England and Wales over 5 million prescriptions were written for liquid preparations of penicillin, at a cost of £2½m., enough to supply every pre-school child in the country with 25 teaspoonsful; and 2¾ million prescriptions for liquid preparations of tetracyclines, at a cost of almost £1m. a year, enough to supply 13 teaspoonsful for every pre-school child in the country – despite the fact that tetracyclines are contraindicated before the age of 6 or 7 because of their effect on the teeth, and because there are alternative antibiotics which are more effective. Innumerable children are given penicillin or other antibiotics for simple skin infections, injuries, bites or trivial accidents, when no antibiotic is needed. It is quite wrong to prescribe an antibiotic just as a placebo to please the parents.

Many children are given so-called 'tonics'. There is no such thing as a tonic; what is given as a 'tonic' is never necessary. Innumerable babies and children are given nose drops for colds, when nose drops are of no value for colds and may do harm. There is no indication for drops for a baby's nose. Yet in one year 1,265,000 prescriptions were written in England and Wales for only four different preparations of nose drops, at a cost of £111,500; they amounted to 19,473 litres (4283 gallons) of nose drops, enough to supply 75 drops for every pre-school child in the country. It is quite wrong to prescribe antibiotics for uncomplicated colds; they have no effect on them. Children are given medicine for influenza, another virus infection; no medicine is necessary or effective. The most that one might give is an aspirin, and that is unnecessary. Innumerable prescriptions for coughs are dispensed; it is hardly ever necessary to prescribe an expectorant for a child, and anyway expectorants are largely useless (with the sole possible exception of iodides), and cough suppressants are usually contraindicated in a child, because a child's cough is so rarely a dry one. It is quite unnecessary to prescribe a cough 'linctus' for a child; yet in one year almost $8\frac{1}{4}$ million prescriptions were written in this country for only seven different paediatric cough linctus preparations, at a cost of £1,325,300; enough was prescribed (769,743 litres, 169,320 gallons) to give 40 teaspoonsful to every pre-school child in the country. Children are given ear drops for otitis media, instead of antibiotics by mouth or injection. I have seen a child with congenital ptosis who had an ointment rubbed on the eyelid daily for over a year, and a child who had had ointment rubbed on the legs for several months because he was a 'late walker'.

Though it is true to say that untold millions of pounds are wasted on unnecessary drugs, whether at home or hospital, I do not wish to suggest that the doctor or hospital spending less on drugs than others is necessarily more efficient; some recently introduced drugs are not only more expensive than previous drugs but also more effective; but it is wrong to prescribe an expensive new drug instead of the less expensive well-established drug just because of some imaginary, hearsay, unproved or marginal advantage over its predecessors, or because of a vague clinical impression.

References

ANON. (1967) Drug warnings and precautions (leading article). *International Medical Digest*, 83, 403.

BRYANT H. (1955) Unprescribed drugs. *Medical Officer*, 7 Oct. 209.

CREERY R.D.G. (1955) Magnesia and alkaline carminatives in infancy. *Brit. Med. J.* 2, 178.

MEYLER L. & PECK H.M. (1968) Drug induced diseases. Amsterdam, Excerpta Medica Foundation.

PROGER S. (1968) *The Medicated Society*. London, Macmillan.

SIDE EFFECTS OF DRUGS (General)

The side effects of drugs are so numerous that it behoves everyone to be fully aware of their frequency. There is probably no drug which is entirely free from at least occasional undesirable side effects. An American study (*International Medical Digest* 1967) found that 300,000 patients are admitted to American hospitals every year for drug-induced illness. One in every twenty patients admitted to the medical wards of Johns Hopkins Hospital, Baltimore, was suffering from the side effects of drugs. It was calculated that over 10 per cent of 1,160 patients in a Belfast hospital on drug therapy suffered from undesired effects. The corresponding figure in Montreal was 18 per cent. In my book, *Common Symptoms of Disease in Children* I have discussed 112 common symptoms and their causes; at least 90 of these symptoms may be due solely to drugs. Because of the importance of these side effects, I have listed the known side effects of drugs used in the treatment of children. It would clearly be impossible to arrange these in order of frequency. Many of the toxic actions listed are rare; but I felt that for reference purposes it would be useful to make the list as comprehensive as possible.

Side effects are due to a wide variety of mechanisms. They may be due to:

overdosage;

suggestion;

susceptibility and hypersensitivity;

superinfection (*e.g.* by moniliasis);

toxicity;

masking effect (*e.g.* corticosteroids masking abdominal pain);

interaction with other drugs: one drug may potentiate another (*e.g.* alcohol and barbiturates); one drug may increase the excretion or metabolism of another drug and therefore make it less effective (*e.g.* sodium bicarbonate increases the excretion of salicylate); a drug may displace another from plasma or tissue protein; a drug may cause electrolyte imbalance and so increase the action of another (potassium loss caused by diuretics may increase the toxicity of digoxin);

drug addiction;

degradation of quality (*e.g.* old tetracycline).

The possible interaction of drugs must always be remembered. For instance, in adult therapeutics it is now well known that monoamine oxidase inhibitors interact with drugs of the ephedrine type. The combination of chloramphenicol and a barbiturate may cause coma. When a child has been receiving phenobarbitone and phenytoin, the withdrawal of phenobarbitone may precipitate acute toxic symptoms from the phenytoin, which may reach a dangerous serum level. The side effects of a drug (*e.g.* drug fever, jaundice) may themselves mimic an existing disease, making the true diagnosis difficult.

If a child has an unusual or severe reaction to a drug, it should be reported to: The Medical Assessor, Committee on Safety of Drugs, Queen Anne's Mansions, Queen Anne's Gate, London SW1.

References

Anon. (1967) Drug interactions. *Drug and Therapeutics Bulletin*, 5, 89.
Anon. (1967) Drug warnings and precautions. *International Medical Digest*, 83, 403.
Anon. (1969) Adverse reactions to drugs (leading article). *Brit. Med. J.* 1, 527.
Beckman H. (1967) *Dilemmas in Drug Therapy*. Chicago, W.B. Saunders.
Hurwitz N. & Wade O.L. (1969) Intensive hospital monitoring of adverse reactions to drugs. *Brit. Med. J.* 1, 531.

SIDE EFFECTS OF INDIVIDUAL DRUGS
(From Illingworth R.S. (1971). *Common Symptoms of Disease in Children*, 3rd ed. Oxford, Blackwell Scientific Publications.)
(With additions.)

Some of the side effects listed could be produced by drugs prescribed only by the hospital doctor or consultant; but the side effects are listed here because the drugs may be taken in the home.

Drugs

Acetaminophen (Paracetamol) – hypoglycaemia, granulopenia.

Acetazolamide (Diamox) – drowsiness, paraesthesiae, excitement, diarrhoea, vomiting, polydipsia, irritability, headaches, vertigo, depression, action on blood, kidney, liver, renal calculus, fever, rash, confusion, melaena, haematuria, glycosuria, fits.

Actinomycin D – action on blood, diarrhoea, rash, alopecia, oral ulcers, intestinal ulceration.

Adrenaline – pallor, sweating, tremor, fainting, nervousness.

Aminophylline – overventilation, fits, haematemesis, anxiety, delirium, coma, fever, respiratory paralysis, dehydration, shock, rashes, headache, death, vomiting, thirst, agitation, restlessness, haematuria.

Amitriptyline (Tryptizol) – drowsiness, dry mouth, constipation, blurring of vision, sweating, pruritus, vertigo, excitement, ataxia, rash, numbness, paraesthesiae, action on blood, tremors, fatigue, weakness, headache, abdominal pain, nausea, vomiting, oedema of face, mouth ulcers, fits, jaundice.

Amphetamine – insomnia, irritability, rash, anorexia, drowsiness, excitability, aggressiveness, jaundice, hyperthermia, dilated pupils, dry mouth, sweating, tremor, paranoia, drug dependence.

Ampicillin (Penbritin) – *see* Penicillin.

Anabolic steroids, *e.g.* Norethandrolone (Nilevar), Methandienone (Dianabol) – jaundice, premature closure of epiphyses, lowered P.B.I., raised serum lipoids.

Anthisan – *see* Antihistamines.

Antihistamines – vertigo, dry mouth, fainting, headache, amblyopia, confusion, frequency of micturition, dysuria, hallucinations, fits, action on blood, drowsiness, irritability, insomnia, urinary retention, tachycardia, gastric disturbance, potentiate barbiturates.

Aspirin – *see* Salicylates.

Atebrin – *see* Mepacrine.

Azathioprine (Imuran) – action on blood, abdominal pain, vomiting, nausea, rash, herpes, pancreatitis, fever, jaundice, amenorrhoea.

Bacitracin – action on kidney, anorexia, nausea, rash. Pain at site of injection.

Barbiturates – rash, drowsiness, irritability, bad behaviour (especially in mentally subnormal child), purpura, hepatosplenomegaly, megaloblastic anaemia, insomnia, nystagmus, poor concentration, Stevens Johnson syndrome, drug dependence. Withdrawal symptoms – fits, tremors, delirium.

Bephenium – nausea, diarrhoea, vomiting.

Betamethazone – *see* Corticosteroids.

Boric acid – red beefy rash, haemorrhages, diarrhoea and vomiting, peripheral circulatory failure, death.

Calcium chloride – gastric irritation.

Capreomycin – action on kidney, deafness, hypocalcaemia, hypokalaemia.

Carbamazepine (Tegretol) – dizziness, vomiting, drowsiness, rash, fits, purpura, Stevens Johnson syndrome, disseminated lupus, diplopia, action on blood, amblyopia, diarrhoea.

Carbenicillin – *see* Penicillin.

Cephalexin – nausea, vomiting, anorexia, abdominal discomfort, super-infection, neutropenia, rash, diarrhoea.

Cephaloridine (Ceporin) – rash, action on kidney, neutropenia, haemolysis, allergy, nausea, vomiting, superinfection, oedema, fever.

Ceporin – *see* Cephaloridine.

Chloramphenicol – Newborn baby – Grey syndrome of failure to thrive, cyanosis, vomiting, irregular respirations, abdominal distension, loose stools, flaccidity, hypothermia, death. – Other children – action on the blood, especially granulopenia, hepatitis, peripheral neuritis, optic neuritis.

Chlordiazepoxide (Librium) – drowsiness, poor memory, overactivity, mania, vertigo, ataxia, extrapyramidal symptoms, hypotension, urinary difficulty, rashes, jaundice, nausea, constipation, action on blood, oedema, vomiting, anorexia, abdominal discomfort.

Chloromycetin – *see* Chloramphenicol.

Chloroquin – retinal changes (maybe delayed for 4–5 years), cataract, burning in mouth, nausea, jaundice, rashes, vomiting, loss of hair, loss of colour of hair, poor accommodation, burning in epigastrium, action on blood, myopathy, photosensitivity.

Chlorothiazide group – potassium loss, allergy, action on blood, vertigo, cramp, pancreatitis, melaena.

Chlorpheniramine (Piriton) – *see* Antihistamines.

Chlorpromazine (Largactil) – *see* Phenothiazines.

Clioquinal (Enterovioform) – neurological symptoms.

Cloxacillin – *see* Penicillin.

Codeine – drying of secretions, collapse of lung if cough productive.

Colistin – deafness, action on kidney, nystagmus, vertigo, paraesthesiae, muscle weakness.

Corticosteroids – sodium retention, mooning of face, Cushing's syndrome, obesity, striae, acne, suppression of pain in infection, increased severity of chickenpox, operative shock, panniculitis, pancreatitis, hyptertension, fits, peptic ulcer, osteoporosis, growth inhibition, diabetes, sudden death, delayed healing, thromboembolic phenomena, cataract, purpura, muscle weakness, thrombocytopenia, dermal atrophy, granulocytosis.

Cortisone – *see* Corticosteroids.

Corticotrophin (ACTH) – same as corticosteroids; more tendency to acne, hyptertension, hirsutism, pigmentation, allergy, less dyspepsia, bruising, striae, osteoporosis.

Cyclophosphamide – action on blood, anorexia, nausea, diarrhoea, vomiting, cystitis, jaundice, headache, intestinal ulceration, alopecia, oral ulcers, myelitis, amenorrhoea.

Cycloserine – neurotoxic, psychoses, fits, action on blood.

Demethylchlortetracycline (Ledermycin) – excessive sunburn, facial oedema, staining of teeth, photosensitivity.

Dexamethasone – *see* Corticosteroids.

Diamox – *see* Acetazolamide.

Diazepam (Valium) – drowsiness, ataxia, nausea, vertigo, depression, acute excitement, hallucinations, diplopia, headache, dysarthria, tremors, rash, action on blood, jaundice.

Diazoxide – hypertrichosis.

Dichlorophen – diarrhoea, rash, abdominal discomfort, vomiting, urticaria.

Digoxin – coupling of the beats, vomiting, oliguria, nausea, bradycardia

Diphenoxylate (Lomotil) – nausea, vomiting, drowsiness, dizziness, rash, insomnia, depression, pruritus, ataxia, nystagmus, pinpoint pupils, deep respirations, coma.

Epanutin – *see* Phenytoin.

Ephedrine – insomnia, pallor, tremor, headache, palpitation, nervousness, nausea, sweating.

Equanil – *see* Meprobamate.

Ergotamine – gangrene, nausea, vomiting, headache, numbness, tingling, chilling of extremities.

Erythromycin – nausea, vomiting, abdominal pain, diarrhoea, rash, jaundice (mainly the estolate), allergy.

Ethacrynic acid – pancreatitis, ventricular fibrillation, electrolyte disturbance.

Ethambutol – rash, gastrointestinal symptoms, retrobulbar neuritis, reduced visual acuity, loss of colour vision.

Ethamivan (Vandid) – convulsions.

Ethionamide – salivation, diarrhoea, vomiting, abdominal pain, liver, mental changes, anorexia, peripheral neuritis, acne, alopecia, photosensitivity.

Ethosuximide (Zarontin) – depression, drowsiness, vomiting, nausea, headache, rash, effect on blood, fatigue, abdominal pain, anorexia, toxic psychosis, disseminated lupus, action on kidney and liver, hiccough, vaginal bleeding, stomatitis.

Fenfluramine – toothgrinding, dyskinesis, diarrhoea, poor concentration, drowsiness, lethargy, nightmares, confusion, withdrawal – agitation.

Flufenamic acid – diarrhoea.

Framycetin – deafness.

Fucidin – *see* Sodium fusidate.

Furadantin – *see* Nitrofurantoin.

Gentamicin – deafness, action on kidney, permanent vestibular damage, alopecia, blurred vision.

Gold – rashes, stomatitis, diarrhoea, hepatitis, albuminuria, action on blood.

Griseofulvin – disseminated lupus, action on blood, kidney, liver, stomach, headache, vertigo, insomnia, peripheral neuritis, poor concentration, photosensitivity, superinfection.

Hyoscine – atropine like action, flushing, drowsiness.

Ibuprofen – dyspepsia.

Imipramine (Tofranil) – jaundice, gynaecomastia, dryness of mucous membranes, tachycardia, sweating, vertigo, glossitis, dysphagia, cold extremities, Parkinsonism, oliguria, insomnia, abdominal pain, tremors, drowsiness, anxiety, rashes, delirium, pruritus, action on blood, impaired accommodation, difficulty in micturition, fits, nausea, postural hypotension, palpitation, dysarthria, sudden falls, giddiness, constipation, irritability, tearfulness, poor concentration.

Imuran – *see* Azathioprine.

Indocid – *see* Indomethacin.

Indomethacin (Indocid) – headaches, drowsiness, vomiting, diarrhoea, nausea, peptic ulcer, confusion, blurred vision, rash, psychological changes, ataxia, jaundice, pancreatitis, asthma, death, corneal and retinal changes, pruritus, vertigo, anorexia, oedema, leucopenia, buccal ulcer, salivary gland enlargement.

Iodides – coryza, acne, gastric disturbance, goitre, swelling of salivary gland, oedema of eyelids.

Iron – constipation, diarrhoea, blackening of teeth and stools, abdominal discomfort. Intramuscular (iron dextran (Imferon), iron sorbitol (Jectifer)) – staining of skin, vomiting, pain, vertigo.

Isoniazid – peripheral neuritis, action on blood, rash, vertigo, excitability, cramp, fits, vomiting, jaundice, albuminuria, gynaecomastia, psychological changes, pancreatitis, disseminated lupus.

Kanamycin – deafness, albuminuria, vertigo, tinnitus, rash, action on blood, amblyopia, paraesthesiae, diarrhoea, superinfection.

Largactil – *see* Chlorpromazine.

Ledermycin – *see* Demethylchlortetracycline.

Librium – *see* Chlordiazepoxide.

Lincomycin – diarrhoea, vomiting, rash, abdominal pain, pruritus, super-infection, muscle pain, rashes, overgrowth of yeasts, jaundice, neutropenia.

Lomotil – *see* Diphenoxylate.

Mefenamic acid – diarrhoea, leucopenia, haemolysis, rash, dyspepsia.

Mellaril – *see* Thioridazine, Phenothiazine.

Mepacrine (Atebrin) – yellow staining of skin, action on blood, psychosis.

Meprobamate (Miltown, Equanil) – depression, Parkinsonism, agitation, ataxia, vomiting, anorexia, vertigo, blurred vision, gastroenteritis, bronchospasm, thirst, frequency, anaphylactoid reaction, drowsiness, rash, action on blood, fever, stomatitis, proctitis, sensitivity reaction, drug dependence. Withdrawal – insomnia, tremors, twitching.

Mepyramine (Anthisan) – *see* Antihistamines.

6-Mercaptopurine – jaundice, action on blood, diarrhoea, vomiting, anorexia, intestinal ulceration, oral ulcers.

Methimazole – action on blood, rash, jaundice, CNS depression or stimulation, fever, arthralgia, pruritus, oedema, hypothryroidism.

Methotrexate – alopecia, vomiting, diarrhoea, oral ulceration, action on blood, nausea, melaena, rash, lung infiltration, jaundice, abdominal pain, renal tubular damage.

Methylphenidate (Ritalin) – tremors, palpitation, anxiety, dyspepsia, headache, rash.

Milontin – *see* Phensuccimide.

Miltown – *see* Meprobamate.

Mogadon – *see* Nitrazepam.

Morphia – vomiting, nausea.

Mysoline – *see* Primidone.

Nalidixic acid (Negram) – vomiting, nausea, haemolysis, anaemia, fits, confusion, paraesthesiae, myalgia, muscle weakness, drowsiness, visual disturbance, diarrhoea, rash, photosensitivity, headache, vertigo, increased intracranial pressure, hypertension, polyarthritis, glycosuria, hyperglycaemia, false positive for urinary reducing substances, jaundice.

Negram – *see* Nalidixic acid.

Neomycin – deafness, albuminuria, steatorrhoea.

Nitrazepam (Mogadon) – drowsiness, ataxia, salivation, lachrymation, bronchial hypersecretion, ataxia, increased appetite.

Nitrofurantoin – discoloration of primary teeth, peripheral neuritis, anaphylaxis, alopecia, jaundice, rash, action on blood, vomiting, nausea, hallucinations, pulmonary infiltration or oedema, pleural effusion, eosinophilia, fever, angioneurotic oedema, muscle pains, chill, alopecia, headache, action on kidney. Haemolysis in presence of glucose 6 phosphate dehydrogenase deficiency.

Nortriptyline – rash, agitation, oedema of eyes and legs, fever, oliguria. Action similar to amitriptyline.

Novobiocin – jaundice, rash, effect on blood, yellow staining of skin.

Nystatin – diarrhoea, abdominal pain.

Oleandomycin – jaundice.

Ospolot – *see* Sulthiame.

PAS (Para-amino salicylic acid, sodium aminosalicylate) – disseminated lupus, vomiting, haemorrhages, rash, gynaecomastia, drowsiness, pulmonary infiltration, jaundice, diarrhoea, thyroid enlargement, thrombocytopenia, abdominal pain, action on kidney, lymphadenopathy, fever, action on blood.

Paracetamol – granulopenia.

Paromomycin – deafness, action on kidney, steatorrhoea, rash, diarrhoea, vomiting, nausea, headache, vertigo, abdominal pain, superinfection.

Penbritin – *see* Ampicillin.

Penicillin – anaphylaxis, diarrhoea when taken by mouth, rashes, arthralgia, polyneuritis, periarteritis, angioneurotic oedema, asthma, effusion into joints, lachrymation, haemolysis, superinfection.

Perphenazine (Fentazin) – *see* Phenothiazine.

Pethidine – vertigo, nausea.

Pheneturide – action on liver, blood, kidney, rash, ataxia, dyspepsia, osteomalacia.

Phenobarbitone – *see* Barbiturates.

Phenothiazine group of tranquillizers [Thioridazine (Melleril), Trifluoperazine (Stelazine), Chlorpromazine (Largactil), Promazine (Sparine), Perphenazine (Fentazin)] – orthostatic hypotension, extrapyramidal symptoms, effect on blood, jaundice, drowsiness, gynaecomastia, pigmentation of retina, corneal opacities, paralysis of accommodation, sweating, catatonia, tremors, rigidity, Parkinsonism, opisthotonos, oculogyric crises, vertigo, fits, rash, headache, poor concentration, constipation, diarrhoea, stomatitis, lactorrhoea, fever, blue-grey colour of skin, photosensitivity.

Phensuccimide (Milontin) – nausea, vertigo, drowsiness, rash, hepatosplenomegaly, haematuria, ataxia, action on blood, disseminated lupus erythematosus.

Phenylazopyridine (Pyridium) – yellow urine.

Phenytoin (Epanutin) – ataxia, gingivitis, vomiting, abdominal discomfort, diplopia, nystagmus, hirsutism, striae, rash, megaloblastic anaemia, hepatosplenomegaly, jaundice, disseminated lupus, Stevens Johnson syndrome, pigmentation, alopecia, albuminuria, drowsiness, tremors, dysarthria, constipation, joint effusion, nausea, anorexia, headache, amblyopia, haematuria, periarteritis, action on blood, pruritus, thinning of hair, adenopathy, arthropathy, osteomalacia.

Piperazine – blurring of vision, paraesthesiae, difficulty in accommodation, vertigo, abdominal pain, rashes, vomiting, ataxia, coma, allergic purpura, tremors, muscle weakness, confusion, inco-ordination, hallucinations, hypotonia, vomiting, precipitation of fits in epileptics, diarrhoea.

Piriton – *see* Chlorpheniramine.

Polymyxin – albuminuria, neurotoxic, fever, rash, ataxia, paraesthesiae, circumoral numbness, pruritus, vertigo, slurred speech, action on kidney.

Ponderax – *see* Fenfluramine.

Prednisone – *see* Corticosteroids.

Primidone (Mysoline) – drowsiness, ataxia, rash, megaloblastic anaemia, disseminated lupus, alopecia, dysarthria, action on blood, vertigo, diplopia, nausea, vomiting, abdominal pain, psychoses, amblyopia, angioneurotic oedema, thinning of hair, nystagmus, osteomalacia, overactivity.

Promazine (Sparine) – *see* Phenothiazine.

Pyopen – *see* Carbenicillin.

Pyrazinamide – action on liver, limb pains.

Pyridium – *see* Phenylazopyridine.

Rifampicin – red urine, sputum, tears; jaundice, rash, drowsiness, dyspepsia, purpura.

Ristocetin – albuminuria, action on blood, thromboses.

Ritalin – *see* Methylphenidate.

Salbutamol – tremors.

Salicylates – overventilation, vomiting, tinnitus, vertigo, deafness, angioneurotic oedema, bleeding by causing hypoprothrombinaemia or thrombocytopenia. Aspirin particles also cause bleeding by direct action on gastric mucosa. Increase of chronic urticaria, angioneurotic oedema.

Sodium fusidate – diarrhoea, vomiting.

Sparine – *see* Promazine, Phenothiazine.

Stelazine – *see* Trifluoperazine, Phenothiazine.

Streptomycin – deafness, ataxia, rash, paraesthesiae, muscle weakness, fever.

Sulphasalazine – nausea, haemolysis, anorexia, vomiting, headache, muscle pain, rash, fever, action on blood.

Sulphonamides – headache, nausea, rash, vertigo, polyneuritis, crystalluria, jaundice, action on blood, drug fever, myopia, photosensitivity, polyarteritis, disseminated lupus, necrotizing angiitis, pancreatitis. Long-acting suphonamides – Stevens Johnson syndrome.

Sulthiame (Ospolot) – overventilation, paraesthesiae, drowsiness, ataxia, albuminuria, confusion, headache, anorexia, action on blood, status epilepticus, renal calculus, blurred vision, dysarthria, photophobia, vertigo, psychotic excitement, loss of weight.

Synacthen – *see* Tetracosactrin.

Tegretol – *see* Carbamazepine.

Testosterone group – jaundice, virilization, acne, premature closure of epiphyses.

Tetanus toxoid – peripheral neuritis, pruritus, erythema around smallpox scar, sweating, urticaria, dysarthria, wheezing.

Tetracyclines – tooth and nail discoloration, enamel hypoplasia, overgrowth of monilia, diarrhoea, anaphylaxis, myopia, jaundice, fever, rash, peptic ulcer, photosensitivity, bulging fontanelle, disseminated lupus, pancreatitis, abdominal pain, glossitis, pruritus, enterocolitis. Given to pregnant woman – inhibition of bone growth and damage of teeth of foetus. Old stocks – Fanconi-like syndrome – oedema, vomiting, nausea, abnormal aminoaciduria, polyuria, polydipsia.

Thiobendazole – dyspepsia, vertigo, headache, pruritus, tinnitus, numbness, hyperglycaemia, xanthopsia, leucopenia.

Thioridazine (Melleril) – *See* Phenothiazine.

Thiouracil – action on blood, disseminated lupus, lymphadenopathy, acne, fever, jaundice, rash.

Thyroxin – heart failure at onset, loss of weight. Overdose – irritability, tachycardia, diarrhoea, advanced skeletal maturation followed by premature closure of epiphyses.

Tofranil – *see* Imipramine.

Tranquillizers and Antidepressants – *see* Phenothiazine group, Chlorpromazine, Meprobamate, Chlordiazepoxide, Methylphenidate, Imipramine.

Triamcinolone – *see* Corticosteroids.

Tridione – *see* Troxidone.

Trifluoperazine (Stelazine) – muscular rigidity, especially face and jaw tremors, extrapyramidal symptoms, coma, diarrhoea, vomiting, constriction of chest.

Trimeprazine (Vallergan) – drowsiness, dry mouth, nasal stuffiness, vertigo, headache, depression, abdominal pain, rash.

Trimethoprim – nausea, action on blood, rash, vomiting, headache, vertigo, diarrhoea, Stevens Johnson syndrome, paraesthesia, emotional upset.

Troxidone – action on blood, nephrotic syndrome, rash, white vision, grand mal, diplopia, hiccoughs, headache, alopecia, jaundice, acne, disseminated lupus, drowsiness, vomiting, abdominal pain, effusion into joints, irritability, angioneurotic oedema, Stevens Johnson syndrome, haematuria, photophobia.

Tryptizol – *see* Amitriptyline.

Valium – *see* Diazepam.

Vancomycin – fever, paraesthesiae, respiratory arrest, deafness, albuminuria, jaundice, action on blood, thromboses, phlebitis, rash, rigor, urticaria, superinfection.

Vandid – *see* Ethamivan.

Vincristine – peripheral neuritis, alopecia, constipation, abdominal pain, ataxia, paraesthesiae, ptosis, pain in fingers, action on blood, oral ulcers, rash, hoarseness, insomnia, jaw pain, headache, pigmentation, diarrhoea, vomiting.

Viomycin – action on liver, kidney, ears. Hypokalaemia, deafness, albuminuria, rashes, electrolyte disturbances.

Viprynium – red stools, nausea, vomiting, diarrhoea, abdominal pain.

Vitamin A excess – periostitis, fractures, hydrocephalus, increased intracranial pressure, hepatosplenomegaly, stomatitis, anorexia, pruritus, oedema of occiput, vomiting, headache, loss of hair, loss of weight.

Vitamin D excess – hypercalcaemia, nephrocalcinosis, polyuria, anorexia.

Vitamin K excess – haemolysis, kernicterus.

Zarontin – *see* Ethosuccimide.

IMMUNIZATION

Triple vaccine: Whooping cough, diphtheria, tetanus

Family doctors and others are likely to become confused by the repeated changes of directive concerning the recommended age for the immuniza-

tion of infants. On the one hand it is desirable to immunize a child as soon
as possible, particularly against pertussis, because almost all deaths and
serious complications from pertussis occur in the first year, and mainly in
the first six months; hence postponement of immunization is a considerable disadvantage. On the other hand, passive antibodies from the mother,
except in the case of pertussis, may interfere with antibody formation by
the baby if immunization is attempted too soon.

There can be no doubt that infants should be immunized against
diphtheria and tetanus. The pertussis component has not proved altogether effective in preventing pertussis, and it is unfortunately that component which is apt to have the most troublesome side effects. Efforts are
being made to improve the efficacy of the pertussis vaccine.

There has been doubt about the wisdom of giving the 'triple' DPT
vaccine to infants who have had fits. The report of the Committee on the
control of infectious diseases (1966) of the American Academy of Pediatrics recommends that in children with 'cerebral damage' immunization
should be postponed until after one year of age, that single rather than
multiple antigens should be used, starting with a small dose of 0·01–0·05
ml. The pertussis antigen should be given last. The doses should be
preceded by aspirin and phenobarbitone. Others (quoted by Illingworth
1968) have expressed the view that it is safe to give the triple vaccine to
infants known to have had convulsions. If a child has a convulsion after
a dose of the triple vaccine, no further dose of the triple vaccine should be
given – though the convulsion may have been no more than a 'febrile fit'.
It would be safe and wise, however, to continue the tetanus toxoid
immunization alone.

Triple vaccine should be given deep subcutaneously or intramuscularly in three doses each of 0·5 ml., either at 4–6 week intervals, commencing at about 6 weeks, or in accordance with the advice of the Department
of Health and Social Security at 3 months, 5 months and 11 months, with
a booster at 5 years. The wider spacing of the injections is thought to
increase the immunity provided.

Measles, rubella, mumps

The principal object of immunizing against measles and mumps is the
prevention of encephalitis. In parts of Africa and elsewhere measles carries
a high mortality, and immunization is therefore important. Girls are
immunized against rubella in order that they will not acquire rubella in
early pregnancy, with consequent risk to the foetus.

The value and safety of measles and rubella vaccine was discussed by Dudgeon (1969). He wrote that 35 million doses of measles vaccine had been given in the United States and elsewhere in the four years preceding his review. The measles vaccine causes a rise of temperature, malaise and upper respiratory tract symptoms in 5–10 per cent. The vaccine has to be reconstituted with sterile water before use.

The rubella vaccine is reconstituted with sterile water and must be used immediately, or at least within an hour of making it up. It is supplied in single-dose vials with a separate ampoule containing 0·5 ml. of diluent. The injection is given subcutaneously. Side effects are unusual, but there may be a slight rise of temperature, mild symptoms suggesting an upper respiratory tract infection, transient rash or rarely arthralgia or polyneuritis. It should be given to girls between the age of 11 and 13.

It is likely that in the near future, a combined vaccine of measles, rubella and mumps will be available.

No live virus vaccine should be given during pregnancy. Measles and poliomyelitis vaccines should not be given at the same time, because one may interfere with the other.

Killed measles and killed poliomyelitis vaccines are now no longer recommended.

Infants are unlikely to acquire measles under the age of 6 months. An infant or child over that age who has been exposed to measles, and who has some other disease making an attack of measles especially undesirable, can be protected by gammaglobulin. If an attack is prevented, the duration of immunity is only a short one, and he will be susceptible in about three months; if he is allowed to develop an attenuated attack, he will have full immunity.

Attenuating dose: 0·25 g. at all ages; within 72 hours of contact.

Prevention under 1 year: 0·25 g.

        1–2 years: 0·5 g.

        3 years or over: 0·75 g.

Live measles vaccine is not normally combined with gammaglobulin. But if a child is malnourished and unwell, gammaglobulin in a dose of 0·6 mg. per lb. will reduce the severity of the reaction from the vaccine.

Live attenuated measles vaccine, subcutaneous or intramuscular, age 13 months – one dose of 0·5 ml.

Rubella vaccine (Cendevax) for girls only, age 11–13 years.

Poliomyelitis

Every child should be protected against poliomyelitis.

Oral poliomyelitis vaccine is now used in Britain instead of the killed vaccine given by injection. The oral vaccine is given at 3 months, 5 months and 11 months (*i.e.* with triple vaccine), with a booster at 5 years and in adolescence, age 15–19 years. The poliomyelitis vaccine is not given within three weeks of vaccination for smallpox.

Smallpox

It is essential that babies should be vaccinated against smallpox if they live in a country in which smallpox is endemic; but questions have been raised about the routine vaccination of babies in countries in which smallpox is rare, such as the United States.

Neff *et al.* (1967) and Lane *et al.* (1969) noted that the last documented case of smallpox in the United States occurred in 1949, and that since then there may have been 111 deaths from vaccination in that country. In 1968, 572 persons in the United States had confirmed smallpox complications, with nine deaths. The morbidity and mortality was highest in infants, with 112 complications and five deaths per million primary vaccinations. They emphasized the need for safer antigens and greater attention to contraindications to vaccination. If vaccination in infancy were shown to protect against encephalitis on revaccination, and if primary vaccination in later years carried a significant risk of encephalitis, this information would help to decide whether the risks of primary vaccination in infancy outweigh the risks of primary vaccination later or of an attack of smallpox if unprotected. It will be remembered that many countries demand recent vaccination before admission of persons from abroad. The imponderables make the decision difficult.

Smallpox vaccination is contraindicated in pregnancy because it may kill the foetus; it is absolutely contraindicated in a child with infantile eczema or other rash; in a child receiving corticosteroids, or having received corticosteroids less than a month previously, or other immuno-suppressants; in a child with agammaglobulinaemia (Brandon 1969). If a child has eczema in the home, his sibling should not be vaccinated, for the eczematous child would be likely to develop generalized vaccinia.

The postponement of vaccination for smallpox into the second year is due to the finding that there is a greater risk of encephalitis in the first year than in the second year. It is calculated (Conybeare 1964, Neff *et al.*

1967) that the risk of complications in England and Wales in the first year is 1 in 18,000, while in the second year it is 1 in 40,000. The need for postponement has not been universally accepted; in Austria, Bavaria and Holland, there was no increased incidence of encephalitis when vaccination was carried out in the first year; but it is now recommended in America that it should be performed in the second year. Nevertheless, in places where smallpox is prevalent, vaccination is carried out immediately after birth – or at least in the first weeks. In Hong Kong, vaccination at 3 days of age is the routine, and 94 per cent 'take' satisfactorily.

The postponement of smallpox vaccination to the second year has been criticized on the grounds that attendances at Child Welfare Clinics are not as high in the second year as in the first year, so that fewer children will be vaccinated. Nevertheless, it is wiser, if possible, to postpone vaccination until the second year.

Prevention of tetanus

After immunizing with the triple vaccine, and after giving the necessary booster or boosters, the question of emergency boosters arises when an injury has occurred. Brindle & Twyman (1962) described four cases of an allergic response after tetanus toxoid. The responses include angioneurotic oedema, urticaria, wheezing, dyspnoea and the Arthus phenomenon. Steigman (1968) wrote that there is a striking correlation between reactions to booster doses and the level of circulating antitoxin; when the antibody level is high, there is a high risk of an allergic reaction. He recommended that emergency booster doses should be given not more frequently than at yearly intervals. A leading article in the *Lancet* (1967) declared that it was unnecessary and unwise to give a booster dose within three years of the previous one. Edsall *et al.* (1967) and Peebles *et al.* (1969) wrote that there is no need for an ordinary booster more often than every 10–12 years, and that after four or more injections protection is adequate for more than 12 years, so that emergency boosters need not be given in that period. In the present state of uncertainty about the matter, I would suggest that when an injury occurs, one should not give a booster if a booster has been given within the last three years.

If an injured child has not been immunized, it is no longer the practice to give tetanus antitoxin (Sharrard 1965, Freeman 1967). The risk of a serious sensitivity reaction is too great, and there have been more deaths from the antitoxin than from tetanus in treated wounds in the same period. Apart from deaths, there have been serious reactions, including serum neuritis, which may be permanent. If a patient has once had tetanus antitoxin, he should never be given another dose, partly because of the great risk of anaphylaxis, and partly because it is useless as it is rapidly excreted.

Sharrard considered that when a wound is clean, with minimal tissue damage sustained in circumstances unlikely to involve contamination with tetanus spores, the wound should be cleaned and sutured (or preferably closed with 'Steristrip'): 0·5 ml. of tetanus toxoid is then administered (as a booster if the patient has been previously immunized; or as a first step to immunizing him for the future, if he has not already been protected).

If there is laceration with tissue damage, and there is a possibility of contamination by tetanus spores, or there is a foreign body, as in a road accident, the wound should be cleaned, dead tissue excised under local or general anaesthetic; the wound is closed, a penicillin injection is given (*e.g.* triplopen), and tetanus toxoid is given. Further penicillin is given daily for 7 days.

If there is an abrasion, a graze, or a penetrating wound of the sole by a nail with a possibility of contamination by tetanus spores, the wound is cleaned with hexachlorophane or chlorhexidine, intramuscular penicillin is given, and tetanus toxoid is administered.

If a wound is heavily contaminated (*e.g.* with manure), it is cleaned, dead tissue excised under general anaesthetic, the wound is left unsutured, and intramuscular penicillin and tetanus toxoid are given.

In all cases the remaining immunizing doses of tetanus toxoid are given subsequently.

It must be remembered that tetanus toxoid given to a previously unimmunized person provides no immediate protection; it is given so that full immunization can be given, in order that if there is a subsequent injury nothing more than a booster of toxoid will be required.

All children should be immunized against tetanus.

If not given as part of triple vaccine, give tetanus toxoid 0·5 or 1 ml. subcutaneously or intramuscularly, followed in 6–12 weeks by a second dose, and 12 months later by a third dose.

Tuberculosis

If it is known that a baby or child will possibly be exposed to tuberculosis, even though the possible source of infection is an adult who is said to have healed tuberculosis, it is essential that the child should be protected by BCG. BCG vaccination is entirely satisfactory in the newborn period.

A tuberculin test is carried out at school on children at the age of eleven, and negative reactors are given BCG. Positive reactors are investigated in order to determine whether there are indications of active tuberculosis and whether the source of the child's infection is in the family.

Typhoid fever

If a child is going to a country in which typhoid fever is endemic, he should be given TAB vaccine. There is no doubt that this protects against typhoid fever, but it is doubtful whether it protects against paratyphoid A and B.

The vaccine is given intradermally (0·1 ml.) in two or preferably three injections at intervals of 4–6 weeks. If necessary, the second dose may be given on return from holiday. If TAB vaccine has been given within three years, one booster dose alone is required. Basic immunity lasts for at least three years, but if travel to infected areas is frequent, a yearly booster dose may be given.

Officially suggested schedule

The following schedule accords with the recommendations of the Department of Health and Social Security:

3 months	diphtheria, pertussis, tetanus, oral poliomyelitis.
5 months	second dose of above.
11 months	third dose of above.
13 months	single dose live attenuated measles vaccine.
15 months	smallpox vaccination.
5 years	diphtheria, tetanus, oral poliomyelitis booster.
10–13 years	BCG if tuberculin negative.
15–19 years, or on leaving school	poliomyelitis vaccine; tetanus toxoid; smallpox vaccination.

The following are paraphrased comments from the Department of Health and Social Security.

The antibody response to diphtheria, pertussis and tetanus may be better if the first dose is postponed to the age of 6 months, with subsequent doses two and six months later respectively; but the disadvantage is that the child will not be immune to pertussis at the age when immunity is most important, namely in the first year of life. It is possible that a severe reaction to pertussis vaccine is more common in the first six months of life than subsequently. Owing to the risk of complications, routine primary vaccination is not advised in childhood after the first two years. An interval of 3–4 weeks should normally be allowed to elapse between the administration of any two live vaccines or between the administration of diphtheria, pertussis, tetanus vaccine and a live vaccine, other than oral poliomyelitis vaccine, whichever is given first. BCG vaccine would be given in the newborn period if there is a possibility of exposure to a contact.

References

ANON. (1967) Tetanus toxoid (leading article). *Lancet*, **2**, 662.

ANON. (1969) Influenza vaccines. *Drug and Therapeutics Bulletin*, **7**, 1.

ANON. (1970) Rubella vaccine. *Drug and Therapeutics Bulletin*, **8**, 59.

ANON. (1970) Holiday typhoid and TAB (leading article). *Brit. Med. J.* **1**, 515.

BRANDON M.L. (1969) Vaccination of patients receiving long term corticosteroid therapy. *J. Am. Med. Ass.* **207**, 1724.

BRINDLE M.J. & TWYMAN D.G. (1962) Allergic responses to tetanus toxoid. *Brit Med. J.* **1**, 1116.

CONYBEARE E.T. (1964) Illness attributed to smallpox vaccination 1951–60. *Monthly Bull. Ministry of Health and Public Health Laboratory Service*, **23**, 126, 150, 182.

DICK J. (1969) Immunisation of children against virus diseases. *Brit. J. Hosp. Med.* **2**, 463.

DUDGEON J.A. (1969) Measles vaccine. *Brit. Med. Bull.* **25**, 153.

DUDGEON J.A. (1969) Rubella vaccine. *Brit. Med. Bull.* **25**, 159.

EDSALL G., ELLIOTT M.W., PEEBLES T.C., LEVINE L. & ELDRED M.D. (1967) Excessive use of tetanus toxoid boosters. *J. Am. Med. Ass.* **202**, 17.

FARDEN D.F. (1967) Unusual reactions to tetanus toxoid. *J. Am. Med. Ass.* **199**, 125.

FREEMAN A.G. (1968) Human tetanus antitoxin. *Brit. Med. J.* **1**, 119.

ILLINGWORTH R.S. (1968) *The Normal Child*. 4th edn. London, Churchill.

LANE J.M. & MILLAR J.D. (1969) Routine childhood vaccination against smallpox reconsidered. *New Engl. J. Med.* **281**, 1220 (see also leading article p. 1241).

LANE J.M., RUBEN F.L., NEFF J.M. & MILLAR J.D. (1969) Complications of smallpox vaccination, 1968. *New Engl. J. Med.* **281**, 1201.

NEFF J.M., LANE J.M., PERT J.H., MOORE R., MILLAR J.D. & HENDERSON S.A. (1967) Complications of smallpox vaccination. *New Engl. J. Med.* **276**, 125.

PEEBLES T.C., LEVINE L., ELDRED M.C. & EDSALL G. (1969) Tetanus toxoid emergency boosters. *New Engl. J. Med.* **280**, 575.

POLK L.D. (1970) Pertussis vaccine. New thoughts on an old vaccine. *Clinical Pediatrics*, **9**, 313.

SHARRARD W.J.W. (1965) The prophylaxis of tetanus. *Prescribers' Journal*, **4**, 120.

STEIGMAN A.J. (1968) Abuse of tetanus toxoid. *J. Pediat.* **72**, 753.

INFANT FEEDING

I have discussed the problems and management of infant feeding in detail elsewhere (Illingworth 1968). Below is a summary of the essential points concerning breast and artificial feeding.

Breast feeding

When the child should first be put to the breast. There is no rule about this. Some mothers feel the desire to put the baby to the breast as soon as he is born, and there is no contraindication to this if the child is fit and not premature. On the other hand, she may wish to rest for twelve hours or so before feeding the baby.

The feeding schedule. A reasonable self-demand schedule is the rational method of feeding the baby in the early weeks. In about two months the child will have chosen a fairly regular schedule, and thereafter the child is fed at regular intervals which have proved to suit him. There is no place for rigidity either way. It will not do the child any harm to cry for a quarter of an hour while his mother is finishing some cooking; but it would be senseless deliberately to keep a child waiting for a specified exact time between feeds, as if all babies were the same.

The doctor must know that a baby who is premature, ill, drowsy, cold or mentally defective cannot be relied upon to demand feeds. It is also important to know that many babies from about 5–10 days after birth demand frequent feeds – up to twelve in the 24 hours. If a baby demands only three feeds in the 24 hours, the breast will remain unemptied for too long and lactation will fail; in such a case the baby should be encouraged to take more frequent feeds.

Prelacteal fluid. In hot weather, sterile boiled water may be given before the milk comes in; otherwise it is better not to give additional fluid because of the risk of introducing infection.

The diet during lactation; drugs in the milk. It is thought by some that if the mother takes onions or pickles, the baby will be upset.

Certain drugs pass through in the breast milk and may affect the baby;

47

they are thiouracil, phenobarbitone, alcohol, bromides, iodides anti-coagulants, and possibly penicillin, ergot, cascara, rhubarb, senna and aloes.

Duration of each feed. All babies are different, and it is easier for babies to obtain milk from some nipples or breasts than others. There can be no rigid rule. Babies obtain most of the milk from a breast in the first three or four minutes. No baby needs more than 10–15 minutes sucking at each breast; if he sucks longer he will merely swallow air and so have 'wind'. The older or more mature baby will need less time than the younger one. The wise mother allows the baby to suck on the first breast until the baby suddenly slows down in his sucking, and on the second until he falls asleep or 'plays'.

It is doubtful whether the time on the breast should be limited in the first two or three days. Some feel that if the baby sucks more than two or three minutes on the first day, he may make the nipple sore. This is uncertain.

The baby should suck from each breast at every feed, for otherwise the breast will remain unemptied too long and lactation will fail.

Emptying the breast. It would be wise for the mother to express the breast after every feed for the first ten days, giving the baby the milk expressed. This helps to avoid overdistension and stimulates the breast to produce more milk.

Twins. The quickest way to feed twins is to feed them simultaneously, with the babies' legs at the mother's side, and the heads propped up on a pillow.

Overdistension of the breast. When the breast of a primipara fills up unusually early or rapidly, at the end of the first day or the beginning of the second, it is wise to give stilboestrol 10 mg. four times a day to slow down the coming in of the milk, discontinuing as soon as congestion is relieved, and following it by manual emptying of the breast until lactation is established. When the breast is already distended, expression should be carried out if it can be done painlessly, and if necessary stilboestrol should be given. The baby should be encouraged to take frequent feeds. If there is severe overdistension, the baby will not be able to obtain the milk and he should not be allowed to try for he will make the nipple sore; the mother is given stilboestrol and sedatives with a breast support, and as soon as congestion is relieved the stilboestrol is discontinued and manual expression is carried out until lactation is established.

Local overdistension of a segment of the breast is relieved by massage towards the nipple.

Sore nipple. The baby is taken off the affected breast, the milk is expressed by hand at every feed time and given to the baby, a greasy preparation (*e.g.* chlorhexidine cream) is applied to the nipple, and the baby is returned to the breast as soon as the nipple is healed.

Blood in the milk. It is probably as well to take the baby off the breast, giving stilboestrol 10 mg. 6-hourly for ten days to stop the milk.

Lactorrhoea. When the milk leaks out of the breast opposite to that on which the baby has begun to suck, or when the breasts leak milk at night when the baby has missed a feed or not had one for a longer time than usual, the mother has to wear a pad of cotton wool to catch the milk.

Insufficiency of milk. It is useless to advise a mother to drink large quantities of fluid when lactating. This will certainly not increase the milk supply and may reduce it. No medicines or food preparations increase the milk supply. The most important way of increasing the milk supply is to empty the breast fully after each feed, giving the baby the milk; the feeds must be sufficiently frequent to stimulate the breast; and the mother should if possible obtain sufficient rest.

When the milk is slow in coming in, nothing but boiled water should be given to the baby until the fifth day, when an artificial feed should be given *after* the breast feeds, the baby being allowed to take as much as he wants (*i.e.* he is given a complementary feed). One should never give a complete bottle feed (supplementary feed) in between the breast feeds, or lactation will fail. The breast must be expressed manually after every feed, the milk being given to the baby.

If there is not sufficient milk by the 14th day, the steps to be taken depend on the quantity of milk which the mother is producing. If she is producing more than half the required quantity, the feed should be made up by complementary feeds. If the mother is not producing half the required quantity ($2\frac{1}{2}$ oz. per lb. per day), it would be wise to stop the breast-feeding altogether, shortening the time on the breast each day until by the end of a week the baby has been taken off the breast.

If the baby has been fully breast-fed for as long as 4–6 weeks, rather

C

than obtaining bottles, teats and the usual equipment for artificial feeding, she may well be advised to wean the baby direct on to thickened feeds.

The irritable baby. If the baby screams when put to the breast, despite there being sufficient milk, it is important to see that his nose is not being obstructed by the mother's breast. He should not be kept waiting for a feed. The problem is that of the first ten days only.

The drowsy baby. Feeds should be offered at regular times, because he may not demand feeds. He should not be kept waiting for feeds, for he may tire himself by crying.

The young baby may go to sleep before he has had sufficient milk, and then awaken in an hour and demand another feed. He will soon get out of this (*e.g.* by about eight weeks) as he matures.

Constipation. Constipation does not occur in breast-fed babies unless they have Hirschsprung's disease, but it is normal for fully breast-fed babies to pass only one stool in several days (up to ten days). No treatment of any kind should be given. It is normal.

Diarrhoea. Diarrhoea is extremely rare in *fully* breast-fed babies. Some breast-fed babies pass as many as 24 stools in the 24 hours; the stools as always are loose; they are often green and contain curds. The baby thrives. No treatment is required. It is normal.

Vomiting. All babies bring some milk up after feeds. At 4–6 weeks, 1 in 150 boys and 1 in 750 girls develop pyloric stenosis. The treatment for this is surgical and *not* medical. The child should be referred immediately to hospital.

The so-called 'pylorospasm' is a myth. There is no justification for giving atropine methyl nitrate or other antispasmodic.

Overfeeding. This is a myth.

Defective weight gain. The treatment depends on the cause. It may be insufficiency of milk, vomiting or overclothing causing fluid loss.

Evening colic. If the diagnosis is correct, it will be relieved by dicyclomine hydrochloride syrup, a teaspoonful before the evening feed. It must be remembered that babies cry because they want to be picked up, or because they are hungry. If a baby stops crying when picked up, he has no significant pain.

Vitamins. If the mother is taking sufficient fruit and greens, there will be no need to give the baby additional Vitamin C. The baby will need additional Vitamin D, in the form of codliver oil (a teaspoonful a day) or adexolin (10 drops a day).

Weaning. There is no rule as to the age at which weaning should be commenced. If it is postponed after about five months, the baby may become difficult about taking new foods. There is much to be said for commencing thickened feeds by four or five months, gradually taking the baby off the breast over the next few weeks.

Thickened feeds consist of puréed meat, vegetables or fruit; soup; cereals; custard; potato mashed with gravy; banana mashed with sugar and milk. Solid foods cannot be given until the baby can chew, *i.e.* 6–7 months in a normal baby.

Artificial feeding

The bottles and teats must be thoroughly washed out immediately after feeds, and then placed in a hypochlorite solution (*e.g.* Milton). Alternatively the bottles and teats may be boiled.

Choice of food. There is nothing to choose between the various dried foods except in price. *It is never necessary to change from one dried food to another to find one which suits the baby – except in the case of the rare metabolic diseases such as galactosaemia or phenylketonuria.* The cheapest foods are those made by Cow and Gate or Glaxo (Ostermilk).

Quantities. The calculated quantity is made up as shown on Table I, and for ease of reference this has been translated into Table II.

When using Cow and Gate, one calculates that the baby will require $1\frac{3}{4}$ measures of the milk powder per lb. (454 g.) per day, a teaspoonful of

TABLE I

Quantity of food for baby, per pound of expected weight per day

	Milk	Sugar	Water
Breast milk	2½ oz. (71 ml.)		
Cow's milk	1¾ oz. (49 ml.)	1 dr. (60 mg.)	¾ oz. (21 ml.)
National Dried Milk, half or full cream	1¾ measures	1 dr. (60 mg.)	2½ oz. (71 ml.)
Full cream Cow and Gate Ostermilk No. 2			
Half cream Cow and Gate Ostermilk No. 1	2½ measures		2½ oz. (71 ml.)
Unsweetened evaporated milk	1½ oz. (42 ml.)	½ dr. (30 mg.)	2½ oz. (71 ml.)

TABLE II

Average quantities for each of the five feeds

Expected weight (or actual weight if greater)	pounds	6 (2·7 kg.)	8 (3·6 kg.)	10 (4·5 kg.)	12 (5·4 kg.)
Breast	oz.	3 (85 ml.)	4 (113 ml.)	5 (142 ml.)	6 (170 ml.)
National Dried Milk, half or full cream, Cow and Gate full cream, Ostermilk No. 2	Milk (meas.)	2½	3½	4½	5
	Sugar (teasp. or dr.)	1 (60 mg.)	1½ (90 mg.)	2 (120 mg.)	2½ (150 gm.)
	Water (oz.)	3 (85 ml.)	4 (113 ml.)	5 (142 ml.)	6 (170 ml.)
Cow and Gate half cream, Ostermilk No. 1	Milk (meas.)	3	4	5	6
	Sugar (teasp. or dr.)	—	—	—	—
	Water (oz.)	3 (85 ml.)	4 (113 ml.)	5 (142 ml.)	6 (170 ml.)
Trufood	Milk (meas.)	2½	3½	5	6
	Sugar (teasp. or dr.)	—	—	—	—
	Water (oz.)	3 (85 ml.)	4 (113 ml.)	5 (142 ml.)	6 (170 ml.)
SMA	Milk (meas.)	3	4	5	6
	Sugar (teasp. or dr.)	—	—	—	—
	Water (oz.)	3 (85 ml.)	4 (113 ml.)	5 (142 ml.)	6 (170 ml.)

Expected weight (or actual weight if greater)	pounds	6 (2·7 kg.)	8 (3·6 kg.)	10 (4·5 kg.)	12 (5·4 kg.)
Evaporated	oz. milk	1 (28 ml.)	1½ (42 ml.)	1¾ (49 ml.)	2 (57 ml.)
	dr. sugar	1 (60 mg.)	1½ (90 mg.)	2 (120 mg.)	2 (120 mg.)
	oz. water	3 (85 ml.)	4 (113 ml.)	5 (142 ml.)	6 (170 ml.)
Fresh cow's milk	oz. milk	2 (57 ml.)	2½ (70 ml.)	3½ (98 ml.)	4½ (127 ml.)
	dr. sugar	1 (60 mg.)	1½ (90 mg.)	2 (120 mg.)	2 (120 mg.)
	oz. water	1 (28 ml.)	1½ (42 ml.)	1½ (42 ml.)	1½ (42 ml.)

sugar per lb. per day, and 2½ oz. (71 ml.) of water per lb. per day (150 ml. per kg.).

It is essential to see that the baby gets enough. Some want more than the calculated quantity, and some less. If he is below the expected weight, because of past underfeeding, the quantity is calculated for the expected weight. This is worked out on the basis of a weight gain of 6 oz. (170 g.) a week in the first three months; *i.e.* at eight weeks his expected weight would be the birth weight $+6\times8 = 48$ oz. (1·36 kg.) over the birth weight.

It is never correct to accept without question a mother's statement that the child is receiving x oz. of Cow and Gate. One has to enquire what she is putting into the x oz. She may be making it up too dilute, in which case the baby may not get enough; or too strong, in which case the baby may suffer from hyperelectrolytaemia and convulsions. There have been many papers in this country, the USA, Japan and elsewhere about the danger of overconcentrated feeds (see references). There is plenty of latitude in infant feeding, and it is entirely correct to make up one measure of Cow and Gate to 1 oz. of water; but one should not make up, say, 4 measures in 1 oz. of water.

Some mothers give overconcentrated feeds because of the idea that a measure holds 1 oz. of water, not understanding that the measure is intended for milk powder and not for water.

It should be noted that prolonged boiling of milk concentrates it and may cause overconcentration of electrolytes by evaporation (Berenberg *et al.* 1969).

The mother must be discouraged from the absurd practice of putting a rusk or biscuit into the bottle. It is likely to block the hole in the teat and may make the child fat by providing excess of cereal. If there is any tendency to excessive weight gain, cereals should be cut down to a minimum. The premature introduction of cereals may be an important cause of obesity.

It is customary, but unnecessary, to warm the feed before giving it to the baby.

There is no need to use half-cream milk except for a premature baby or one which has had diarrhoea. Full-cream milk is used from the beginning.

Additional vitamins. Vitamin D is added by the manufacturers of the dried milks and cereals. There is no need to give additional Vitamin D. Vitamin C should, however, be given.

Weaning. There is no rule about the age at which weaning should be commenced. It can begin at 3 or 4 weeks, if desired. I normally recommend the addition of thickened feeds when the baby reaches 10 lb. or so. The thickened feeds are *not* put into the bottle, but are given by spoon and cup, or by cup alone.

The teat. By far the commonest source of difficulty in artificial feeding is too small a hole in the teat. If the hole is too small, the baby takes too long over the feed and swallows air, and so has 'wind' and may vomit. No feed should take more than 10–15 minutes. It is common to find that feeds are taking 45–60 minutes. It is wrong to rely on the maker's statement that the hole in the teat is small or large. The patency and size of the hole should be tested before every feed, by inverting the bottle with the milk in and teat in place; without any shaking, the milk should almost pour out – not in drops which can be counted. The hole readily becomes blocked by milk powder or lumps, and so it must be tested before every feed. If the teat is of rubber, the hole can be enlarged by inserting a needle in a cork, making the needle red-hot, and so enlarging the hole.

Excessive wind. This is almost always due to the hole in the teat being too small. It may be due to allowing the baby to suck on an empty bottle or on a teat which has flattened because there is a vacuum in the bottle, the baby having sucked the air out.

It is useless to give carminatives or 'dill-water'. The cause of excessive wind should be sought.

Vomiting and colic. The cause should be sought.

Constipation. This may be due to giving insufficient fluid, especially in hot weather. Constipation can often be corrected by adding more sugar, or by giving puréed fruit, such as prunes. Only when this has been tried and has failed should milk of magnesia be given.

Diarrhoea. This may be due to excess of sugar or to gastroenteritis.

Defective weight gain. This may be due to insufficiency of milk or water, to vomiting, diarrhoea or any infection.

Excessive weight gain. This may be due to the premature introduction of cereals, such as rusks or other starchy foods. A baby who is gaining weight excessively should not have more than 1 pint of milk a day, and should be weaned on to thickened feeds with careful limitation of carbohydrate.

Refusal of the bottle. This is dealt with by feeding the baby with cup and spoon.

References

ANON. (1970) Feeds which infants will not tolerate (leading article). *Brit. Med. J.* 4, 515.

BERENBERG W., MANDELL F. & FELLERS F.X. (1969) Hazards of skimmed milk, unboiled or boiled. *Pediatrics*, 44, 734.

ILLINGWORTH R.S. (1968) *The Normal Child.* 4th edn. London, Churchill.

SIMPSON H. & O'DUFFY J. (1967) Need for clarity in infant feeding instructions. *Brit. Med. J.* 3, 537.

SKINNER A.L. (1967) Water depletion associated with improperly constituted powdered milk formulas. *Pediatrics*, 35, 625.

BEHAVIOUR PROBLEMS: GENERAL COMMENTS

In my book *The Normal Child: Some problems of the first five years and their treatment*, and to some extent in *The Normal School Child: His Problems Physical and Emotional*, I have discussed in detail the basis of behaviour problems, their prevention and treatment, dealing first with the general principles and then with each behaviour problem in turn. I do not wish to overlap too much with what has been written there, but it is impossible to discuss in this book the management of the many common behaviour problems seen by the family doctor in the home, without referring to some of the conclusions reached in my previous books. I have therefore summarized below the main causes of behaviour problems and their management.

A child's behaviour depends on the interaction of prenatal, natal and postnatal factors and environment with his developing personality and needs. His personality is partly inherited and partly the product of his environment, particularly in the home, and later in his school and neighbourhood. Parents who themselves had a happy childhood and are warm, loving, understanding and tolerant, with a good sense of humour, are much more likely to have happy, loving children than those parents who unfortunately do not possess these qualities.

A child's physical health inevitably affects his emotional health, and therefore one basic requirement is good health, good food, warmth and comfort, and the prevention of disease – all problems concerning the family doctor.

The child's basic emotional needs include above all the need for love and security, wise, loving discipline and the gradual acquisition of independence. He needs not only to be loved but to feel loved, wanted and accepted – particularly when he is feeling irritable and bad-tempered, or behaving badly; for children need loving most when they are being most unlovable. This does not mean giving him everything that he wants. Every child has to learn to accept a No; he has to learn that he cannot have everything that he wants. Overindulgence is a potent cause of insecurity and therefore of bad behaviour. It does mean that there must be no favouritism whatever, no ridicule, no sarcasm, no unfavourable comparison with a sibling, no derogation, no criticism, no threat to withhold love as a punishment for disobedience, no talking to others in front of a child about his shortcomings. If a child is to be happy, the home must be happy – free from friction between mother and father, free from constant friction between parent and child. Perpetual naggings and reprimands do nothing but harm. In some homes every day is one long series of remonstrances. Children constantly need encouragement rather than discouragement, praise rather than disapproval, implantation of good behaviour and good manners rather than punishment for bad behaviour; children, like animals, learn far more effectively by the positive approach of praise and reward than by the negative approach of overstrictness and disapproval.

Children are rendered thoroughly insecure by punishment and intolerance. Punishment is nearly always wrong; it nearly always represents nothing more than loss of temper on the parents' part. Children are punished and reprimanded for acts which are in no way wrong, for actions which they have copied from their parents, or which arise from the subconscious mind and which for that or some other reason they could not possibly avoid; for instance, most bedwetters are punished by their parents, and it hardly seems rational to punish a child for something which he does in his sleep. Children are rendered insecure if their parents are intolerant – perhaps because of fatigue, ill health or worry, or because of their ignorance of a child's normal psychological needs and development – for example, the normal negativism of the 1–3-year-old, the normal aggressiveness and quarrelsomeness of the 3–6-year-old, or the negativism, emotionalism and awkwardness of the child at puberty. They are rendered insecure by frequent moves from house to house, school to school, or by prolonged separation from their parents.

Children may feel insecure if too much is expected of them; if the effort to inculcate good manners is made long before they are ready for it; if more is expected of them at school than their intellectual endowment will permit; if the parents react by criticism and disapproval to any negative comment in the school report; if they are expected to concentrate more on their homework than their level of intelligence will make possible; if there is overstrictness, overindulgence, failure to allow the development of independence when they are ready for it; or if there is teasing at home or school on account of obesity, spots on the face, awkwardness and clumsiness, dirty or unsuitable clothes, or any other shortcoming. Jealousy is a form of insecurity; it represents in the child's mind the feeling that he is not loved as much as he needs to be, or as much as he used to be, or that he is not as important or as much wanted as he used to be. All children need constantly to be certain that they are loved, wanted, accepted and important; unkindness, criticism, ridicule and disapproval do nothing but harm.

Insecurity is at the root of a wide variety of behaviour problems, either alone or in conjunction with other factors; the symptoms include excessive fears, timidity, shyness or weeping; clinging to the mother, excessive nailbiting and thumbsucking; excessive jealousy, aggressiveness, destructiveness, showing off, night terrors or masturbation; and in some children bedwetting, faecal incontinence, hostility, stuttering, tics, head banging, stealing or truancy.

The management of insecurity depends on the cause. The family doctor, knowing the family, is in the best possible position to guide the parents. He knows their personality and the personality of their children. He may decide that part of the problem is the mother's fatigue; the treatment of the child's behaviour problem may consist of iron medicine for the mother's iron deficiency anaemia, or the treatment of her menorrhagia, or the referral of the mother to hospital for her thyrotoxicosis. He may find that the child's behaviour problems are related to his difficulty in reading, which requires investigation by an educational psychologist; that his truancy results from the teachers' regarding the child's bad writing as due to naughtiness and carelessness, when in fact it is due to minimal cerebral palsy or clumsiness which he cannot help or to his being consistently bottom of the class – and that a psychologist should assess the child's ability by IQ testing in order to decide whether he is in the most suitable type of school. He may find that the child's problems are due to bullying at school; and he may get the mother to arrange judo classes so that the child can acquire confidence to deal with the bully. He may decide to get in touch with the school medical officer, in order to determine whether there are problems in the school which can be remedied or he may advise the parents to see the teacher in order to try to find a joint answer to the child's difficulties. He may seek the help of a health visitor. The family doctor must know what causes insecurity and its resulting problems. It does not help the parent to be told that 'it's just his nerves', or that 'he'll grow out of it'. The treatment is not a matter of prescribing sedatives, tranquillizers or antidepressants; it is a matter of knowledge of the normal and normal psychological needs and development, and then of the use of common sense.

References

ILLINGWORTH R.S. (1964) *The Normal School Child: His Problems Physical and Emotional*. London, Heinemann.
ILLINGWORTH R.S. (1968) *The Normal Child*. 4th edn. London, Churchill.

ANTIBIOTICS

Introduction

The frequent appearance of new antibiotics, after a long succession of previous antibiotics, each with the statement that it is highly effective for a long list of infections, leaves the hospital and doctor and the general practitioner in a state of confusion. The result is frequently that the doctor turns to a new antibiotic, usually very expensive, only to find, after time for proper trials to be conducted and experience to be gained, that it is less effective than the older well-established antibiotics and has dangerous side effects.

In this section I have tried to state the present position as to the choice of antibiotics, and my recommendations are made in the full knowledge that some of them may change with time.

Antibiotics not indicated

Antibiotics are *not* indicated for the following conditions:
colds;
cough following colds, other than penumonia;
asthma, or acute bronchitis, unless it is complicated by pneumonia;
small pustules in the newborn;
boils;
the common dysentery; mild salmonella infections;
gastroenteritis; non-specific diarrhoea;
infectious mononucleosis;
sore throats, until proved to be streptococcal.

Antibiotic synergism

There is some evidence that the following drugs exert a synergistic action when prescribed together:
penicillin and streptomycin (subacute bacterial endocarditis);
pencillin and kanamycin;
streptomycin and tetracycline (brucellosis);
colistin and sulphadimidine (proteus infections);
colistin or polymyxin with chloramphenicol or tetracycline;
trimethoprim and sulphamethoxazole.

Antibiotic antagonism

It may be unwise to combine a bactericidal drug with a bacteriostatic one. The following are examples of bacteriostatic drugs: Chloramphenicol, erythromycin, oleandomycin, sulphonamides, tetracycline, novobiocin, lincomycin, fusidic acid. The following are bactericidal: Penicillin, streptomycin, neomycin, cephalosporins, polymyxin, nalidixic acid, kanamycin, vancomycin, colistin, gentamicin.

It follows that penicillin should *not* be prescribed along with such drugs as tetracycline or erythromycin. It should not be combined with fusidic acid. In addition, it is thought that penicillin should not be prescribed with vancomycin; chloramphenicol should not be prescribed with tetracycline; tetracycline should not be combined with the cephalosporins or chloramphenicol. Penicillin and sulphonamides should not normally be prescribed together except for meningococcal infections. The cephalosporins should not be prescribed with tetracyline, chloramphenicol, fusidic acid or erythromycin. Neither vancomycin nor nalidixic acid should be prescribed with bacteriostatic drugs (*Drug and Therapeutics Bulletin*, 1968).

The evidence for some of these examples of antagonism is in some cases doubtful; but in the present state of our knowledge it would be unwise to ignore them.

Cross-resistance

There are now so many antibiotics, many of them close relatives, that it is difficult to remember when to expect cross-resistance to occur.

There is usually cross-resistance between erythromycin, lincomycin and oleandomycin.

There is usually cross-resistance in the neomycin, gentamycin, kanamycin group.

Wise and unwise guessing in antibiotic therapy

When a newborn baby becomes ill with an infection, he should be sent to hospital. Amongst other things, he may have pyogenic meningitis – a condition not usually associated with neck stiffness in this age group.

It is wrong to prescribe an antibiotic when meningitis is suspected. The child should be sent to hospital immediately, in order that a lumbar puncture can be carried out, the infecting organism determined, and the correct treatment prescribed. Unwise antibiotic therapy in the home reduces the child's chances of survival from pyogenic meningitis. If one does have to guess the appropriate treatment, before the laboratory can report the organism and its sensitivities, it would be wise to prescribe kanamycin and ampicillin together, because they would cover nearly all the likely organisms.

When a child has pneumonia, it is safe to prescribe benzyl penicillin without laboratory help, though there are organisms such as mycoplasma which would not respond.

It is safe to guess the cause of otitis media and prescribe penicillin. (Some doctors prefer ampicillin, because of the possibility that the infection is due to haemophilus influenzae.)

It is unwise to guess the correct treatment for urinary tract infection, partly because of the great difficulty in making an accurate diagnosis in the home (with the difficulty of obtaining a really clean specimen and getting it examined promptly), and partly because it is important that the causative organism should be isolated and its sensitivities determined, in order that the appropriate antibiotic can be prescribed. Furthermore, a urinary tract infection should be properly investigated even in a first attack, and all cases should therefore be referred to a hospital consultant.

Failure of antibiotics

When an infection fails to respond to an antibiotic, the following are the possible reasons:

   (i) organism insensitive, virus infection;
  (ii) wrong diagnosis;
 (iii) wrong drug;
 (iv) wrong dose;
  (v) drug given by wrong route;
 (vi) drug resistance;
(vii) drug antagonism;
(viii) mixed infection;
 (ix) presence of pus;
  (x) drug not taken long enough;
 (xi) drug not taken frequently enough;
(xii) drug not taken at all.

Infections and available antibiotics

This table is fairly complete, not because many of these infections would be treated at home, but because in many cases treatment would be instituted in hospital and continued at home.

Infection	Antibiotic of choice	Other antibiotics to which the organism is usually sensitive
Haemolytic streptococcus	Benzyl penicillin	Sulphadimidine. Erythromycin. Lincomycin, Fusidic acid. Polymyxin. Cloramphenicol. Tetracycline. (As the haemolytic streptococcus is almost invariably sensitive to penicillin, there is rarely indication for the above.)
Pneumococcus	Benzyl penicillin	Erythromycin. Sulphadimidine. Lincomycin. Polymyxin. Tetracycline. Chloramphenicol. (As the pneumococcus is almost invariably sensitive to penicillin, there is rarely indication for the above.)
Staphylococcus. Penicillin resistant	Cloxacillin	Methicillin. Erythromycin. Cephalosporins. Lincomycin. Fusidic acid. Kanamycin. Gentamicin. Neomycin. Trimethoprim. Tetracycline. Chloramphenicol. Vancomycin. Ristocetin. Bacitracin (infants only). Polymyxin.
Staphylococci. Penicillin sensitive	Benzyl penicillin	Ampicillin, Cloxacillin. Erythromycin. Cephalosporins. Fusidic acid. Vancomycin. Ristocetin. Bacitracin (infants only). Trimethoprim. Tetracycline. Lincomycin. Chloramphenicol. Sulphonamides. Neomycin. Kanamycin. Gentamicin. (There is rarely an indication for any of the above if the organism is sensitive to penicillin.)
E.coli	Sulphadimidine (Urinary tract)	Urinary tract – Ampicillin. Nitrofurantoin. Nalidixic acid. Gentamicin. Kanamycin. Trimethoprim. Others – Chloramphenicol. Tetracycline. Streptomycin. Neomycin. Polymyxin. Cephalosporins. Colistin. Vancomycin.
Proteus	Ampicillin	Colistin. Ampicillin. Streptomycin. Neomycin. Gentamicin. Kanamycin. Polymixin. Trimethoprim. Novobiocin. Chloramphenicol. Cephalosporins. Sulphadimidine.
Pseudomonas pyocyaneus	Carbenicillin	Neomycin. Kanamycin. Gentamicin. Colistin. Polymyxin. Streptomycin.
Streptococcus faecalis	Ampicillin	Streptomycin. Tetracycline. Chloramphenicol. Polymyxin. Kanamycin. Vancomycin.
Haemophilus influenzae	Ampicillin	Chloramphenicol (for meningitis only). Cloxacillin. Penicillin. Streptomycin. Tetracycline. Polymyxin. Sulphadimidine. Cephalosporins. Erythromycin.
Meningococcus	Sulphadimidine and Penicillin	
Pertussis	Uncertain? None	Ampicillin. Kanamycin. Neomycin. Tetracycline.

Infection	Antibiotic of choice	Other antibiotics to which the organism is usually sensitive
Salmonella	None* (except severe infections)	Ampicillin. Kanamycin. Gentamicin. Chloramphenicol. Tetracycline. Paromomycin. Cephalosporin. Neomycin. Polymyxin.
Shigella	None**	Sulphadimidine. Ampicillin. Gentamicin. Neomycin. Kanamycin. Cephalosporins. Tetracycline. Streptomycin.
Monilia	Nystatin	Amphotericin.
Diphtheria	Erythromycin	Cephalosporins.
Cl. Welchii	? Ampicillin	Erythromycin. Kanamycin. Penicillin. Tetracycline. Streptomycin. Chloramphenicol. Polymyxin.
Aerobacter aerogenes	?	Colistin. Gentamicin. Neomycin. Streptomycin. Tetracycline.
Brucella	Tetracycline	Streptomycin. Kanamycin. Chloramphenicol.
Actinomycosis	Penicillin	Neomycin. Sulphadimidine. Tetracycline. Chloramphenicol. Erythromycin.
Klebsiella pneumoniae (Friedlander)	? Ampicillin	Cephalosporins, Gentamicin. Kanamycin. Chloramphenicol. Streptomycin + Sulphadimidine. Polymyxin. Sulphadimidine.
Tuberculosis	Isoniazid with Streptomycin or PAS	Rifampicin. Ethionamide. Ethambutol, etc. (These should be prescribed only by a chest physician or other consultant.)

* Except for typhoid fever, paratyphoid A. B. or C.
** Except for severe illness.

NOTES ABOUT INDIVIDUAL ANTIBIOTICS

I have written about penicillin first, as it is by far the most useful of all antibiotics, and I have followed with notes on the other antibiotics in alphabetical order.

Penicillins

There is a bewildering number of penicillins, and the situation is confused by the numerous trade names for the same preparation. In fact for ordinary use the National Formulary Procaine Penicillin injection or the combined rapid and long-acting preparation 'Triplopen' are the usual preparations for injection for such conditions as pneumonia, streptococcal tonsillitis or otitis media. For oral use, phenoxymethyl penicillin is satisfactory. When a child is ill, it is wise to commence the treatment by an intramuscular injection and then to continue by the oral route.

The synthetic penicillins have important advantages and disadvantages, and because of the latter and their expense they should not be used routinely when a penicillin is required. Ampicillin is useful because of its broad spectrum, which includes H.Influenzae (and is therefore appropriate for otitis media, which is often associated with that organism), and gram negative bacteria such as *E. coli*, and is therefore helpful for urinary tract infections. One drawback of ampicillin is the frequency of rashes. Shapiro *et al.* (1969) found that a rash developed in 9·5 per cent of 422 patients receiving ampicillin, and 4·5 per cent of 622 receiving other penicillins. Ampicillin has largely replaced tetracycline, because it covers the same organisms, is more effective, and does not stain the teeth. Cloxacillin is used for penicillin resistant staphylococcal infections, as is methacillin; the latter can be given by intramuscular injection only. *The synthetic penicillins are less effective for penicillin sensitive staphylococcal infections than the ordinary penicillins (benzyl penicillin or phenoxymethyl penicillin) – and for this reason the newer preparations should not be used routinely for such infections.*

Carbenicillin, given intravenously or intramuscularly only, is used for pseudomonas infections; it must be made up freshly for each patient. The injection may be painful.

If one penicillin causes an allergic reaction, it is almost certain that the others will have the same effect.

If a child is allergic to penicillin, one should give erythromycin (in preference), lincomycin, trimethoprim, fusidic acid or perhaps cephalexin, but some patients who are allergic to penicillin are also allergic to the cephalosporins.

The four main types of sensitivity to penicillin are:
(1) anaphylaxis – immediate;
(2) delayed – fever, urticaria, effusion into joints, enlargement of the lymph nodes and spleen, as in serum sickness;
(3) contact dermatitis;
(4) sensitivity rash.
Each year there are 100–300 deaths from penicillin sensitivity in the USA.
One should always ask about penicillin allergy before prescribing the drug.

A penicillin sensitive child should wear a Medic-Alert bracelet or necklet, as a warning to doctors who are about to treat him: they are obtained from the Medic-Alert Foundation, 43a Wigmore Street, London W1.

The following list gives official and trade names of penicillins.

Official name	*Trade name*
Ampicillin	Penbritin
Benzathine penicillin	Penidural
Benzyl penicillin	Solupen, Crystapen G
Benzyl penicillin potassium	Cathopen, Eskacillin
Benzyl penicillin sodium	Crystapen (inj.)
Benzyl penicillin B.P.	Falopen
Carbenicillin	Pyopen
Cloxacillin	Orbenin
Methicillin	Celbenin
Penicillin G	Crystapen G
Phenethicillin potassium BP	Broxil
Phenoxymethyl penicillin	Penicillin V
	Crystapen V
	Distaquaine V etc.
	Pedipacs V Cil K
	Penicals
	Stabillin VK
	Campocillin VK
	V Cil K
Procaine penicillin	Distaquaine G
	Duracillin AS
	Prostabilin

Procaine penicillin
    with benzyl penicillin   } Triplopen
    and benethamine penicillin

Propicillin potassium BP   Ultrapen, Brocillin

The choice of penicillins is so wide and confusing that I would advise the family doctor to make his choice from the following only:

Oral   – phenoxymethyl penicillin NF.

           – benzyl penicillin for prophylaxis only (*e.g.* rheumatic fever).

           – ampicillin where indicated.

Injection – Triplopen – once per day (intramuscularly) or procaine penicillin injection BP

           – benzyl penicillin.

	Route	Number per day	Newborn	1 year	7 years	Puberty
Benzyl penicillin	IM	2	15 mg./kg.	150 mg. (250,000 u)	300 mg.	600 mg.
Ampicillin	Mouth or IM	4	62·5 mg.	125 mg.	250 mg.	500 mg.
Phenoxymethyl penicillin	Mouth	4	62·5 mg.	125 mg.	250 mg.	500 mg.
Procaine penicillin injection BP	IM	1	150 mg.	300 mg.	600 mg.	1 g.
Triplopen	IM	1 every day (? every 2 days)	0·6 ml.	1·3 ml.	1·3 ml.	1·3 ml.

Bacitracin

This is used mainly for local application to the skin (*e.g.* otitis externa, impetigo), but sensitivity is apt to occur.

It may be used on the advice of a paediatrician for penicillin resistant staphylococci in infants only, given intramuscularly in a dose of 1,000 units/kg./day at 8–12 hour intervals; and 900 units/kg./day for premature babies.

Cephalosporins

These include:
Cephaloridine,
Cephalothin,
Cephalexin.

The latter alone can be given by mouth. These drugs are useful for penicillin resistant staphylococcal infections, unless they are resistant to cloxacillin and methicillin; and they are useful for urinary tract infections including those due to bacillus proteus. They cover the same range of organisms as ampicillin and tetracycline, and include streptococci, *E.coli*, salmonella and shigella. Cephalexin is relatively non-toxic. There may be cross sensitivity to penicillin, so that it is not necessarily safe to use these drugs for a child who is allergic to penicillin.

The cephalosporins are expensive and should not be used if other drugs are available, *i.e.* without firm pharmacological and bacteriological indications.

Preparations for intramuscular use must be freshly prepared for each patient.

Trade names for cephalexin are Keflex or Ceporex;
for cephaloridine, Ceporin.

Cephaloridine must be given by intramuscular injection only.

Cephalexin is given by mouth. Dose: newborn 15 mg./kg.

$$\left.\begin{array}{l} \text{1–11 months 125 mg.} \\ \text{1 year 250 mg.} \\ \text{7 years 500 mg.} \\ \text{Puberty 500 mg.} \end{array}\right\} \text{q.d.}$$

Chloramphenicol (trade name: Chloromycetin)

Chloramphenicol should virtually never be prescribed in general practice. Its main use is for typhoid fever and possibly influenzal meningitis. It is of doubtful value in pertussis, and being so dangerous it should not be used for that infection. It should not be used for the common salmonella infections, partly because of the risk of side effects, and partly because antibiotics merely prolong the carrier state without shortening the illness. There is no excuse for prescribing chloramphenicol for respiratory infections.

The principal danger of chloramphenicol is a blood dyscrasia. Best (1967) wrote that 408 fatalities had been reported to the American Medical Association Registry between 1953 and 1964. Fatalities were by no means always related to the dosage, 10 per cent of the deaths occurring after a dose of less than 8 mg./kg./day. A blood dyscrasia may occur during therapy, in which case the total dose is important, and recovery is the rule; or in a delayed form after cessation of therapy, unrelated to the total dosage and usually fatal.

It is tragic to cause a fatal aplastic anaemia by prescribing a drug unnecessarily – when other safer drugs would have been equally effective.

Colistin (trade name: Colomycin)

The family doctor is unlikely to prescribe this drug himself. It is used mainly for pseudomonas infections, but also for certain gram negative bacteria. It is nephrotoxic, and may cause troublesome paraesthesiae. It is given by injection only.

Erythromycin (trade names: Erythrocin, Ilotycin, Ilosone), Oleandomycin

These should be used only rarely in general practice, and only when the infecting organism has been shown to be sensitive to them and insensitive to other antibiotics.

Erythromycin is probably the drug of choice for diphtheria; it covers the same organisms as penicillin, but is not as effective as cloxacillin or methicillin for penicillin resistant staphylococci. It is certainly not as effective as penicillin for the treatment of streptococcal or pneumococcal infections. It should not be used for longer than 5–7 days, because resistance to it rapidly develops. The erythromycin estolate is more apt than other preparations to cause toxic hepatitis, so that other preparations of erythromycin are recommended. It is often wise to combine it with another antibiotic to reduce the risk of the development of resistance.

Oleandomycin has no advantage over erythromycin, is more expensive and is less effective. Triacetyloleandomycin is less effective than erythromycin against streptococci and pneumococci; it may cause hepatitis.

Erythromycin can be given by mouth or intramuscularly:

1st year	12 mg./kg.	
1 year	125 mg.	q.d.
7 years	250 mg.	
Puberty	500 mg.	

Fusidic acid (trade name: Fucidin): sodium fusidate

Fusidic acid, given by mouth, is effective against penicillin insensitive staphylococci and its use may be justified for children who are allergic to penicillin when the organism is sensitive to fusidic acid; but erythromycin is the drug of choice under these circumstances. The drug can also be used for the treatment of diphtheria.

Doses, by mouth:

1st year	50 mg./kg./daily, divided into 3 doses
1–5 years	250 mg./kg./daily, divided into 3 doses
5–12 years	500 mg./kg./daily, divided into 3 doses
Puberty	750 mg./kg./daily, divided into 3 doses

Neomycin (trade names: Neomin, Nivemycin, etc.), Kanamycin (trade names: Kantrex, Kannasym), Gentamicin (trade names: Cidomycin, Genticin), Paromomycin, Framycetin Group

These drugs are strongly ototoxic and nephrotoxic, and should only be used for definite indications. It is doubtful whether they should be used by the family doctor, because, with the exception of neomycin and framycetin used locally, they would be used only for an ill child who needs hospital treatment. Neomycin and framycetin are sometimes used locally for skin infections, but skin sensitization may occur. Framycetin is closely related to neomycin.

There is little to choose between neomycin, kanamycin, gentamycin and paromomycin, though kanamycin is the least toxic; it is given intramuscularly only, mainly for infections in the newborn, covering infections by gram positive cocci, *E.coli*, some strains of *B.proteus* and pseudomonas, and haemophilus influenzae. Cloxacillin is preferable for pencillin resistant staphylococci, and colistin or polymixin B for *B.proteus* and pseudomonas infections.

Gentamicin covers the same organisms. If a child becomes allergic to one of this group (*e.g.* neomycin) he is likely to be allergic to the others.

	Route	Number per day	Newborn	1–11 mths.	1 yr.	7 yrs.	Puberty
Gentamycin	IM	2	Avoid	1 mg./kg.	10 mg.	20 mg.	40 mg.
Kanamycin	IM	2	2·5 mg./kg.	7·5 mg./kg.	75 mg.	200 mg.	500 mg.
Neomycin	Mouth	4	12 mg./kg.	12 mg./kg.	125 mg.	250 mg.	500 mg.

Novobiocin (trade names: Albamycin, Cathomycin)

This has a similar range to penicillin but is less effective. Resistance to it rapidly develops, and so it is wise to combine it with another drug. It could be used for penicillin resistant staphylococci, but cloxacillin is preferable. It is apt to be toxic.

Streptomycin, Lincomycin (trade names: Lincocin, Mycivin), Clindomycin (trade name: Dalacin C)

Streptomycin belongs to the same group as kanamycin and neomycin, and is similarly ototoxic and nephrotoxic. It is used for tuberculosis.

Lincomycin covers the same infections as erythromycin, but has no advantages over it; it could be used for streptococcal, pneumococcal, staphylococcal infections and for diphtheria, but other drugs are preferable (*e.g.* cloxacillin for penicillin resistant staphylococci). Cross-resistance to erythromycin occurs. It could be used for children allergic to penicillin. It is sometimes used in hospital for the treatment of osteitis.

Clindomycin is a new analogue of lincomycin; organisms resistant to lincomycin will also be resistant to clindomycin. The two antibiotics are effective against the same organisms, and both are relatively non-toxic, the only untoward side effects being occasional diarrhoea or vomiting. They may both be used for streptococcal or staphylococcal infections in children who are allergic to penicillin. For prolonged treatment, as for osteitis, clindomycin should be combined with another antibiotic in order to reduce the risk of the development of resistance.

Clindomycin should be given in doses of 8–16 mg./kg./day in 3–4 divided doses.

Sulphonamides

There are numerous sulphonamides, but sulphadimidine is the one most commonly used. There is no advantage in using the more expensive preparations (*e.g.* sulphafurazole or urolucosil). The main indication for sulphonamide treatment is meningococcal or urinary tract infection. Sulphonamides are unlikely now to be used for dysentery infections. Sulphasalazine is confined to the treatment of ulcerative colitis. Sulphamethoxazole is used in conjunction with trimethoprim (Septrin, Bactrim) for the treatment of urinary tract and other infections.

There is no virtue at all in combining sulphonamides (*e.g.* Sulphatriad); the combination is more expensive than sulphadimidine used alone. The combination was originally devised with the idea that it would reduce the risk of renal colic; the solubility and safety of sulphadimidine is such that the combination has no advantages.

It is unwise to prescribe sulphadimidine in the newborn period, because it competes with bilirubin for binding to the plasma proteins and therefore may lead to kernicterus.

Long-acting sulphonamides (*e.g.* sulphamethoxypyridazine) are not recommended because of the risk of the Stevens Johnson syndrome.

Dose of sulphadimidine by mouth:

Newborn avoid
1 year   250 mg. ⎫
7 years   500 mg. ⎬ q.d.
Puberty   1 g.   ⎭

Official and trade names of sulphonamides are listed below.

Official name	*Trade name*
Sulphadimidine	Sulphamethazine
Sulphafurazole	Gantrisin
Sulphamethizole	Urolucosil
Sulphamethoxazole	Gantanol
Sulphamethoxypyridazine	Lederkyn
	Midicel
Sulphaphenazole	Orisulf
Sulphasalazine	Salazopyrin
Sulphathiazole, sulphadiazine, sulphamerazine	Sulphatriad
Sulphathiazole, sulphadiazine, sulphadimidine with streptomycin	Streptotriad
Succinyl sulphathiazole	Sulfasuxidine

Tetracyclines

There are several derivatives of the earlier tetracyclines,
lymetetracycline,
demethylchlortetracycline (Ledermycin),
solitetracycline,
methacycline,
clomocycline,
but there is no evidence that they are better in antimicrobial activity, absorption or freedom from gastrointestinal side effects. Lymetetracycline has one advantage – it is more soluble and therefore useful for intramuscular injection. New derivatives are normally more expensive, and there is no reason to use them unless they offer new advantages (*Drug and Therapeutics Bulletin* 1967).

Paediatricians are now most reluctant to use any tetracyclines before the age of 6 because they stain children's teeth so badly. The tetracyclines react with calcium to form a tetracycline calcium orthophosphate, which is deposited in bone and teeth. Staining of the teeth of the foetus occurs after the 14th week *in utero*. Even a five-day course can lead to permanent staining. The permanent teeth may be stained when tetracycline is given any time after birth.* It is said that oxytetracycline stains less than other derivatives (*Drug and Therapeutics Bulletin* 1967). Stewart (1968) found

---

* Staining occurs especially in the first six years, after which the risk is less, because the permanent and deciduous teeth have fully calcified. Even after that age, prolonged treatment by tetracycline may cause staining of teeth and nails.

that 55 per cent of 464 first permanent molar teeth removed between 7 and 15 years of age for caries had at least one deposit of tetracycline.

Tetracyclines not only stain the teeth; they may cause enamel hypoplasia and deformity of the cusps, while they increase the incidence of dental caries.

There is no point in changing from one tetracycline to another, because there is cross-resistance between them. Most hospital staphylococci are now resistant to them.

There is no point in prescribing a combined preparation of tetracycline and nystatin or amphoteracin with the idea of preventing candidiasis.

If one is compelled to use a tetracycline because there is no other antibiotic to which the organism is sensitive, one would use oxytetracycline, as it is the cheapest and it has not been established that other preparations are more effective. Whenever possible, one would use a different antibiotic because of the effect on the teeth and because they are less effective than other antibiotics. I know of no indication for the use of tetracyclines in a newborn infant.

MacCracken *et al.* (1970) summarized the position as follows: 'Tetracyclines are generally more expensive, always more toxic and usually less effective than penicillin or erythromycin.'

Official and trade names of tetracyclines are:

Official name	*Trade name*
Chlortetracycline	Aureomycin
Clomocycline	Megachlor
Demethylchlortetracycline	Ledermycin
Lymecycline	Armyl, Mucomycin, Tetralysal
Methacycline	Rondomycin
Oxytetracycline	Terramycin, Imperacin, Clinimycin
Tetracycline with oleandomycin	Sigmamycin
Tetracycline	Achromycin
	Ambramycin
	Tetracyn
	Tetrex
	Totomycin
	Tetrachel
	Steclin
	Clinitetrin
Tetracycline with amphoteracin	Mysteclin

Trimethoprim

Trimethoprim in combination with sulphamethoxazole (Septrin, Bactrim) is a new preparation which is of use for urinary tract and staphylococcal infections, and possibly for chronic infections of the respiratory tract and typhoid fever. The two drugs act in synergism. It is used for the treatment of infections resistant to other antibiotics but sensitive to sulphonamides. It is expensive and should only be used for organisms proved bacteriologically to be sensitive to it and insensitive to other drugs. So far there has been no satisfactory controlled trial, so that it has not been shown to be superior to other drugs for routine use in urinary tract infection.

It could be used for children allergic to penicillin if the organism is insensitive to erythromycin, and sensitive to trimethoprim.

	Route	Number per day	Newborn	1 yr.	7 yrs.	Puberty
Trimethoprim with sulphamethoxazole	Mouth	2	Avoid	40 mg.	80 mg.	160 mg.

Vancomycin, Ristocetin

These are given intravenously only. They cover the same organisms as penicillin but are less effective. They could be used for penicillin-resistant staphylococci but are apt to be toxic.

References

ANON. (1962) The choice of systemic antimicrobial drugs. *Drug and Therapeutics Bulletin*, 1, 17.

ANON. (1965) Cephaloridine. *Drug and Therapeutics Bulletin*, 3, 5.

ANON. (1966) Warning against long acting sulphonamides. *Drug and Therapeutics Bulletin*, 4, 13.

ANON. (1967) Old and new tetracyclines. *Drug and Therapeutics Bulletin*, 5, 77.

ANON. (1967) Tetracyclines stain children's teeth. *Drug and Therapeutics Bulletin*, 5, 61.

ANON. (1968) Interaction between antimicrobial drugs. *Drug and Therapeutics Bulletin*, 6, 49.

ANON. (1968) Penicillin allergy and purified penicillin. *Drug and Therapeutics Bulletin*, 6, 9.

ANON. (1968) Symposium on antimicrobial therapy. *Pediatric Clinics of North America*, 15, 1–298.

ANON. (1969) Neomycin and framycetin in topical preparations. *Drug and Therapeutics Bulletin*, 7, 81.

ANON. (1970) Clindamycin. Dalacin C. *Drug and Therapeutics Bulletin*, 8, 67.

BEST W.R. (1967) Choramphenicol-associated blood dyscrasias. *J.A.M.A.* **201**, 99.

EYKYN S.J. & PHILLIPS I. (1969) Advances in antibiotics. *Practitioner*, **203**, 510.

MACCRACKEN G.H., EICHENWALD H.F. & NELSON J.D. (1970) Tetracyclines. *J. Pediat.* **76**, 802.

SHAPIRO S., SISKIND V., SLONE D., LEWIS G.P. & JICK H. (1969) Drug rash with ampicillin and other penicillins. *Lancet*, **2**, 969.

SMITH H. (1969) *Antibiotics in Clinical Practice*. London, Pitman.

STEWART D.J. (1968) Tetracyclines – their presence in children's teeth. *Brit. Dental J.* **1**, 318.

Part 2
The Treatment of Individual Symptoms and Diseases

ABDOMINAL PAIN

I have discussed elsewhere the numerous causes of abdominal pain in children (Illingworth 1971), and it is obvious that the treatment must depend on the cause. The recurrent pain and vomiting in many affected children seems to be a variant of the periodic syndrome, which in turn is probably a manifestation of migraine (see p. 201). In about 94 per cent of children with recurrent central abdominal pain, no organic cause can be found; but organic disease must always be looked for; many children have been thought to have psychogenic abdominal pain when in fact they have a hydronephrosis or peptic ulcer. The history may reveal psychological factors, in the form of insecurity (p. 55), and the doctor will conclude that they are at least a major cause of the symptom. He is likely to refer the child to hospital in order to eliminate organic disease, and then try to deal with the causes of the insecurity. One must not conclude that a symptom in a child (or adult) is entirely of psychological origin just because one cannot find evidence of organic disease; the diagnosis must be based on the elimination of organic disease together with positive signs of psychological disturbance; and it is always as well to follow the patient up in order to ensure that no underlying organic disease reveals itself with the passage of time.

Having decided that the pains are of psychological origin, the family doctor, having done his best with regard to any discoverable causes of insecurity, will advise the parents to pay as little attention to the complaints as possible. The mother who keeps the child off school, puts him to bed, rubs his abdomen and gives him warm drinks each time he complains of a pain, is asking him to continue to have pains and to have worse ones. If the father constantly complains of his gastric discomfort in the child's hearing, it would not be surprising if the child had to complain of pain. It often happens that when the parents are satisfied that there is no organic disease, the child's symptoms assume less importance in the minds of the parents and gradually disappear. They may persist in some children, continuing into adult life as recurrent pains or else as overt migraine.

Anticholinergic or antispasmodic drugs are not of value in treating these children. In fact no medicine helps. Laxatives are to be avoided, being useless for alleviation of the symptom and possibly harmful; sedatives, tranquillizers and antidepressants should not be prescribed.

Reference

ILLINGWORTH R.S. (1971) *Common Symptoms of Disease in Children*. 3rd edn. Oxford, Blackwell.

ACNE

There are probably three components of acne – excessive secretion of sebum, obstruction of the outflow of sebum and inflammation. Acne is related not only to puberty but to drugs – notably corticosteroids, iodides and bromides. It is said that troxidone, codliver oil, chloral, quinine and thiouracil may sometimes cause it.

There is at present no method of reducing the secretion of sebum. Obstruction to the outflow may be prevented by:

(1) soap and water; soap containing sulphur and salicylic acid, used three times a day or more, may help;

(2) one per cent centrimide lotion three times a day;

(3) sulphurated potash and zinc lotion (BNF) applied twice a day and left on overnight;

(4) three per cent sulphur and resorcin in Lassar's paste – especially for the chest and back, left on at night;

(5) abrasion by 'Brasivol' ointment in increasing strength. This is an abrasive in three grades; it is rubbed into the skin for half a minute, left on for five minutes and then washed off; not all dermatologists consider abrasives to be useful);

(6) ultraviolet light once a week, to cause desquamation.

It is unwise to squeeze out the comedones with the finger nails, and still more unwise to scratch them, for scarring may result. A comedo extractor should be used.

For infections, tetracycline (250 mg. q.d.), erythromycin or ampicillin should be used. It is thought by some that a prolonged course of tetracycline in low dosage (e.g. 250 mg. per day) may be valuable even if there is no gross infection. Drugs causing acne should be discontinued.

There is no place for a special diet.

References

ANON. (1966) Management of acne vulgaris. *Drug and Therapeutics Bulletin*, 4, 49.
SNEDDON I. (1963) Acne vulgaris. *Prescribers' Journal*, 3, 50.

ADENOIDS

When a child develops nasal speech, persistent snoring, has recurrent otitis media, mouthbreathing due to postnasal obstruction, or has a persistent postnasal discharge causing a cough at night, he should be examined by an ear, nose and throat specialist, and if the above symptoms are ascribed to adenoids, the adenoids should be removed.

If a child has any speech defect, especially if the speech is nasal, the operation should only be performed after consultation with an expert, because it could make the speech worse.

There is no justification for removing the tonsils at the same time unless there are special indications for tonsillectomy.

AGGRESSIVENESS

See *Quarrelsomeness*.

ALLERGIC RHINITIS

In this section I shall refer only to perennial allergic rhinitis, and not to hay fever. The steps to be taken to prevent dust in the case of the asthmatic child are discussed on p. 86 in the section on asthma. They are no less important for the child with allergic rhinitis. It is not usually possible to find the allergen, and the remarks about the lack of value of skin testing and hyposensitization made on p. 88 apply equally to children with allergic rhinitis. It is a difficult condition to prevent and treat.

Nasal drops should not be used. They may themselves cause rhinitis; they have a secondary congestant action following the decongestion; and it is said that they may damage the cilia. If any drops are used (and I advise against the use of nose drops), the safest would be $\frac{1}{2}$ per cent ephedrine in normal saline.

There is no place for corticosteroids. I know of no therapy which helps these children. The possibility that polypi may develop must be remembered, so that the opinion of the ear, nose and throat specialist may have to be sought. It is said that children with allergic rhinitis are more likely than others to become sensitive to aspirin.

ALVEOLAR FRENUM

This fold of tissue under the upper lip sometimes extends as far as the gum margin. If one sees this in a newborn baby, the question arises as to whether it will cause malposition of the teeth. It does not usually, but it may separate the incisor teeth. In the case of the baby or toddler, no treatment is required. After that age, one would consult the orthodontist if in doubt. He may operate when the child is 6 or 7 years old, but not before.

AMMONIA DERMATITIS

See *Nappy Rash*

ANAEMIA

The treatment of anaemia must depend on the cause, and before embarking on treatment it is wise to have the blood examined by the haematologist, having first referred the child to a paediatrician. Amongst other things, it is important to eliminate gastrointestinal haemorrhage, leukaemia, and the effect of drugs on the bone marrow. Conditions which are associated with a low haemoglobin, and which demand a correct diagnosis so that the appropriate treatment can be given, include rickets, cretinism and lead poisoning. In an African child, sickle cell anaemia has to be eliminated.

A prematurely born baby who has not been given additional iron is likely to become anaemic in the second six months of life, and a guess that the child is suffering from iron deficiency is likely to be a safe one. The family doctor is likely to guess at the same diagnosis when an older pre-school child becomes gradually anaemic without any acute onset of illness.

I frequently see confusion with regard to normal haemoglobin values. I have seen numerous children treated over many months with iron medicine for completely non-existent anaemia, because of failure to recognize the normality of the haemoglobin.

The following figures show the mean and the range of normality for the haemoglobin in full-term babies.

Age	Mean (g. per cent)	Range of normal (g. per cent)
1 day	19·5	14·5–24·5
2 weeks	16·5	—
2 weeks to 3 months	14·0	10·7–17·3
3 months to 5 months	12·2	9·9–14·6
6 months to 11 months	11·8	—
1 year	11·2	10·0–12·0
2 years	11·5	10·0–12·0
3 years	12·5	
5 years	12·6	
6–10 years	12·9	
11–13 years	13·4	
14 years	15·0	

It is particularly important to note the range of normal, especially in the first year, before prescribing iron.

The best treatment for iron deficiency anaemia is ferrous sulphate. The dose for a baby would be 60 mg. twice a day. At five years a reasonable dose would be 180 mg. twice a day. There is no advantage in other more expensive preparations. Ferrous sulphate is the cheapest; it is well absorbed and hardly ever causes gastrointestinal disturbance in a child. There is no evidence that other preparations are any better; there is evidence that several of them are not as good.

D

One avoids intramuscular injections of iron in children (iron dextran, Imferon) because of the possible dangers (serious sensitivity reaction, staining of the skin), and because an intramuscular injection is unpleasant for the child. One gives it only in exceptional cases in which the iron deficiency anaemia fails to respond to the oral preparation and one can be sure that the drug has been given: in these cases one must be sure that one's diagnosis of iron deficiency anaemia is correct, and hospital investigation would be essential.

Having prescribed the ferrous sulphate, it is essential to follow the child up in order to make sure that the blood count shows a satisfactory response, and in order to be sure that no relapse occurs.

Preparations

Iron should be prescribed as ferrous sulphate and not as a trade name, because ferrous sulphate prescribed as such is usually considerably cheaper.

In the BNF mixture there are 60 mg. in 5 ml. The BNF ferrous sulphate tablet is 200 mg.

There is no advantage in prescribing other preparations of iron which are more expensive and often less effective.

Dose:

BNF mixture of ferrous sulphate Up to 1 year – up to 5 ml. t.d.

                                             1–5 years – up to 10 ml. t.d.

BNF tablets   6–12 years – 200 mg. b.d.

ANAL FISSURE

This may be the result of constipation, in which case that must be treated. The local application of lignocaine ointment NF three times a day should be sufficient to relieve the pain and allow the fissure to heal. Other local anaesthetic ointments are better avoided, because they are more apt to sensitize the skin. If an anal fissure after the above treatment fails to heal, the child should be referred to a paediatric surgeon.

ANAPHYLAXIS

The common causes of anaphylaxis are:
(1) tetanus antitoxin as a prophylactic. This should not be used;
(2) penicillin.

If there is immediate anaphylaxis, a tourniquet may be applied to delay absorption from the injected site, but care must be taken not to forget it and leave it on too long. The child should then be given adrenaline: 1 in 1,000 0·12 ml., if a baby; 0·25 ml., if age 1–5; 0·5 ml., if older, intramuscularly. After insertion of the needle, the plunger should be withdrawn to make sure that the needle is not in a vein.

An intramuscular injection of diphenhydramine (Benadryl) 1 mg./kg. (up to a maximum of 50 mg.) may be given, and the child sent to hospital immediately. Corticosteroids may be given there, but they have no immediate action.

ANGIOMA

See *Naevi*.

ANTRUM INFECTION

When a child has a persistent bilateral purulent nasal discharge or a purulent postnasal discharge, it is a safe guess that he has an antrum infection. A unilateral discharge would suggest a foreign body in the nose. When the clinical diagnosis of antrum infection is made, the best treatment is penicillin for not less than ten days. Ideally, a nose swab would be taken prior to instituting treatment, in case the organism is a penicillin resistant staphylococcus. I would give oral phenoxymethyl penicillin if the parents could be relied upon to give it regularly. Only if that failed would the child be referred to a consultant for advice.

When a small child has a persistent antrum infection, one must remember that another member of the household may possibly have the same infection and may be keeping it going.

Most children with bronchiectasis and many with fibrocystic disease of the pancreas have a chronic antrum infection. In either case the antrum infection is difficult to treat because of the chest infection. The chest infection keeps the antrum infection going, and the antrum infection maintains the chest infection. The help of a paediatrician and otolaryngologist is needed.

APPETITE

Loss of appetite during an acute illness is treated by attention to the acute illness. A poor appetite in a well child never calls for medicine. The causes of anorexia have been fully discussed elsewhere (Illingworth 1968). Basically a poor appetite is due to the following causes.

(1) A small physical build, the child taking after the mother or father. Small build may be related to low birth weight – especially in a child who was small in relation to the duration of gestation. The smaller the child at birth the smaller he usually is in later years of childhood. The child may be small because of congenital heart disease, severe asthma or other condition. Whatever the cause, the small child needs less food than the big child, and so may cause anxiety because of what his parents term a 'poor appetite'.

(2) The child's normal ego and negativism. Children normally go through a stage of negativism between 1 and 3, as their ego develops. They characteristically want to do the opposite of what they are asked to do, and attempts to force them to do anything, to eat, go to sleep or use the pottie, are likely to lead to the opposite of the effect desired. At the same time they like to attract attention, to create a fuss and anxiety, and if they can get the whole house revolving around their eating, sleeping or bowels, they will love it. Mothers readily convey their anxiety about the child's appetite by trying to persuade him to eat, coaxing him, offering him bribes (sweets, money, etc.) if he will eat, threatening punishment if he will not eat, or smacking him – and so he refuses.

(3) Giving food between meals. Many mothers are so concerned about

the child's appetite that they offer him constant snacks between meals. I have seen toddlers with food refusal having as many as twenty-five meals a day. Large amounts of milk remove the appetite for other foods; milk should be limited to a pint a day.

(4) Food-forcing. This may be due to anxiety because the child is an only one, or was regarded as delicate, or because the mother is concerned about the normal falling off in weight gain in the second half of the first year – with an associated falling off of the appetite; or because of the mother's overanxiety for other reasons. The toddler normally dawdles with his food – seeing no reason to hurry. This may be interpreted by the mother as lack of appetite. Whatever the cause of her anxiety, she is worried, tries to make the child eat more, and so he refuses – because of his normal ego and the normal negativism from 1 to 3. Determined efforts to make a child eat inevitably lead to food refusal.

(5) Conditioning. When the mother tries to force the child to eat, threatens punishment if he will not eat, or smacks him for not eating, the child learns to associate mealtimes and food with discomfort – and becomes conditioned against food, developing a poor appetite as a result. A mother told me that her boy always began to cry when he saw that a meal was ready. This sort of conditioning is difficult to treat.

No medicine is required for anorexia. It is essential to know what the mother is worried about and what she is doing to try to get the child to eat. It should be explained that *it is never necessary to try to make any child eat. Efforts to do so always lead to food refusal.* The mother should show no anxiety whatsoever about what the child eats. There should be absolutely no persuasion, no praise, no rewards. Eating is normal and there is no reason to praise him for it. As long as a child is being difficult, he should have nothing between meals, however hungry he is. The parents must know that no child starves because he is not persuaded to eat; the child's poor appetite is due to food-forcing (except in the case of the child of small build). If the food refusal and food forcing have been going on for a long time, one must not expect immediate results from the treatment outlined above.

Reference

ILLINGWORTH R.S. (1968) *The Normal Child.* 4th edn. London, Churchill.

ASPHYXIA OF THE NEWBORN

The essential treatment is to see that there is an airway – by aspirating mucus and other material by a mucus catheter. In hospital intubation is performed, so that aspiration can be more effective, and, if necessary, oxygen can be given under controlled pressure. If the child is not breathing after clearing the airway, mouth-to-mouth resuscitation is the best method to use in the home, holding the chin and head back with one hand, and applying pressure to the abdomen with the other hand, while mouth-to-mouth insufflation is carried out.

Drugs are of doubtful value. If the mother had been given morphia or pethidine, nalorphine (Lethidrone) 0·25 mg. IM may help.

It is more doubtful whether nikethamide (Coramine) or ethamivan (Vandid) placed on the tongue, are of any value. No other drug should be given. The most important treatment consists of ensuring that there is an airway and, if necessary, applying artificial respiration.

ASTHMA

Prevention

There are three main components of asthma – allergic, psychological and infective. These three interact, and if one can deal effectively with one of them, the asthma may be relieved.

Allergic factors

It is essential to enquire about possible allergens, though in my experience, perhaps because of insufficient care in taking the history, it is unusual to determine the specific cause for the attacks. Nevertheless, even if one cannot determine the specific allergens, one must attempt to reduce exposure to allergic substances to which the child may well become sensitive in the future. It is unwise, for instance, to have dogs, cats, birds or other pets in the house. If an asthmatic child is particularly attached to a household pet, removal of the animal may well cause emotional distress; I would therefore advise that when the animal dies it should not be replaced.

If any item of food precipitates an attack, that food should be avoided. If a child has a strong dislike for any particular food, one should think of the possibility that he is allergic to it.

Below are suggestions for reduction of allergens.

Keep dust down by daily use of damp cloth.

Pillow – should be Dunlopillo.

Mattress – preferably Dunlopillo; or enclose the mattress in a plastic envelope and seal it.

No eiderdown – not even kapok.

Bedspread – plain cotton or synthetic fibre.

Blankets – cotton preferable to wool. Wash frequently.

Stuffed toys – discard if possible, unless all rubber.

Carpet – avoid if possible. Linoleum is best cover for floor.

Curtains – wash each week if possible.

Venetian blind – avoid.

Clothes in cupboard – keep to a minimum.

Wool clothes should not be worn.

Whole room – vacuum clean once a week.

Walls, ceiling, woodwork, floors – keep clean. Wash woodwork weekly. Wash walls as often as reasonably possible. Damp areas on walls or ceiling must be dealt with.

Pictures – remove.

Furniture – remove dust by damp cloth.

Bed – clean with damp cloth, including springs.

Soft chairs – remove. No upholstered furniture.

Bookcase – remove.

Pets – exclude from the house if possible; avoid having pet animals or birds.

Windows and doors – closed except at night.

Child should dress and undress in another room.

Rest of house – as dust-free as possible.

Central heating – forced hot air type undesirable.

Hay fever – keep window closed at night.

All this may sound excessive; but if the asthma is severe it is well worthwhile for the parents to do their best to reduce the allergens in the child's bedroom. In advocating these steps one must make it clear that one does not expect to cure the asthma by doing this, but that one is trying to prevent the child becoming sensitive to the dust and other allergens in the future.

The value of hyposensitizations is a matter of opinion. Johnstone & Dutton (1968) carried out a controlled trial with 105 children suffering from perennial asthma, given hyposensitization, and 105 controls, given an inert substance. 130 were followed up to the age of 16 years. 72 per cent of the treated children and 22 per cent of the controls were free from asthma at the time of follow-up. In any such trial it is essential to see that treated and control children were in all ways comparable and were chosen blindly or by random sampling. The doctor assessing the results should certainly not know whether the children seen on follow-up had received the active or inactive substance. On the other hand Forgacs & Swan (1968) in a controlled trial with house dust allergy found no advantage in hyposensitization. Fontana, Holt & Mainland in a five-year follow-up of 25 treated and 26 controls (given an inert substance) found that hyposensitization was of no value. In the ensuing discussion it was argued that the antigen used may have been unsatisfactory, that it was given in the wrong way or to unsuitable patients, or that the material used was of poor quality. Other studies have failed to provide evidence that hyposensitization has helped. Peterson (1968) in a review of the subject concluded that 'there is no overwhelming evidence that allergic patients are being deprived of a major therapeutic approach if they are not subjected to repeated injections of the offending allergens. Most of the evidence in favour of desensitization is anecdotal.'

I may be wrong in not favouring skin testing and subsequent hyposensitization, and I do not deny that an occasional child may be helped by it. Jerome Glaser (1969) wrote that a positive skin test does not indicate clinical sensitivity, and that a negative test does not exclude it; a positive test may indicate: (*a*) present clinical sensitivity; (*b*) past sensitivity; (*c*) potential sensitivity. Hyposensitization is unpleasant for the child, demanding a considerable number of pricks, unless one of the 'depot' preparations is used. I disliked the 20–30 injections for the five months preceding the hay fever season; the ever-present itching papule at the site of the previous injection was annoying; and having personally experienced and seen dangerous and alarming reactions to hyposensitization with ordinary aqueous preparations (for hay fever), despite all care with the dosage, I would not myself risk using one of the longer-acting emulsions of grass pollen proteins in mineral oil. These require about 3 injections at monthly intervals, whereas the ordinary preparations require 20 or more. It is feared that there is a remote possibility of a breakdown of the emulsion, which would lead to an overdose. The oil might cause a chronic inflammatory reaction, sterile abscess or cyst. The United States Food and Drug administration will not allow the unrestricted sale of emulsified extracts, but grants a permit to individual practitioners only.

If a severe reaction does occur after an injection of hay fever vaccine, of whatever kind, one would give 1 in 1,000 adrenaline immediately, and apply a tourniquet (see *Anaphylaxis*, p. 83). For such a reaction immediate hospital admission would be required.

If one is able to determine the allergen, it may be possible to avoid exposure to it or to prevent an asthmatic attack, if exposure cannot be avoided. I saw a boy who developed asthma on Fridays only; it became obvious that he was sensitive to dog hair, and that on Fridays he visited his grandmother who had a dog; as soon as he came into contact with the dog he began to wheeze. The problem was dealt with not by hyposensitization, but by giving a small dose of corticosteroid early on Friday morning, well before the visit. A better alternative would be disodium cromoglycate.

Disodium cromoglycate (Intal) has no effect on an attack of asthma, and this should be explained to the parents, who otherwise will be apt to increase the dose if an attack occurs, or else be disappointed that it does not relieve the child. It is supposed to block the result of the antigen antibody reaction and so to prevent the attacks. It is given in a spincap insufflator, morning, midday and last thing at night. 'Intal compound' includes a small amount of isoprenaline because it was thought that the dry powder might irritate the mucosa; the amount is small and safe, but the cromoglycate can be supplied without the isoprenaline if it is so desired. There have been numerous favourable reports, and very few contrary views, on its efficacy. In my experience it has been highly successful in preventing attacks in most (but not all) children. It can be used by a child of 5 or older – and sometimes by a younger child if intelligent and sensible.

I have never been able to convince myself that other drugs are useful in the prevention of asthma. I doubt whether ephedrine helps; it would be given in a dose of 8 mg. twice a day in a pre-school child and 25 mg. twice a day in an older child. Neither have I been impressed by the prophylactic value of the xanthine derivatives, theophylline and aminophylline. Some favour a combination of theophylline, ephedrine and phenobarbitone, sold under the trade name of Tedral or Franol (½ tablet at 6 years three times a day) or choline theophyllinate (Choledyl) 50 mg. at 1 year three times a day, or 100 mg. at 7 years three times a day.

This latter preparation was regarded as the best of the xanthine preparations (*Drug and Therapeutics Bulletin* 1967). These preparations have the drawback that they may cause sleeplessness and abdominal discomfort, and that, being diuretics, they may have a drying action on the bronchial secretions and make the asthma worse. As I have said, I think that they are of doubtful value.

Corticosteroids have an important part to play in the treatment of severe chronic asthma, when other measures have failed. I would recommend that they should only be given under specialist supervision, and all the possible side effects of corticosteroids should be borne in mind. In particular, prolonged use is likely to cause stunting of growth, itself a result of severe asthma. It has been suggested, but not proved, that the use of ACTH 10–60 units daily, or a long-acting preparation tetracosactrin (Synacthen) may avoid this stunting; but intermittent dosage of prednisolone, given three or four days a week instead of daily, is less likely to be complicated by undesirable side effects than daily corticosteroids and probably does not cause stunting of growth. The smallest possible dosage of prednisolone should be given; for instance, 5–10 mg. once a day on 3 or 4 days a week may be sufficient to keep the child clear from asthma. I personally prefer to give prednisolone, because it is given by mouth, rather than ACTH or tetracosactrin. If all other treatments fail, and the alternative is severe chronic disability, it would be wrong to withhold corticosteroids. It has still to be determined whether the best treatment is ACTH or intermittent corticosteroids by mouth. It is certainly reasonable to give a maintenance dose of corticosteroid 3 or 4 times a week if all other methods fail, including disodium cromoglycate. The alternative is to allow the child to be a dwarfed respiratory cripple; but I doubt whether one is ever justified in giving so much corticosteroid that the child develops a marked Cushingoid appearance. There is a real risk of drug dependence and drug addiction. The effect of giving a placebo is well worth trying in a child who is steroid-dependent. Other children have become aerosol-dependent and are in considerable danger as a result. I feel that corticosteroids may be useful to stop an attack, so that disodium cromoglycate can then be given to prevent further attacks. The corticosteroid is discontinued as soon as the cromoglycate has been started.

When a child is receiving corticosteroids, the effect of stress, in the way of infection or trauma including surgical procedures, must not be forgotten; the dose of corticosteroid should be doubled. Even if the child is not taking corticosteroids at the time, but has taken them in the last

6–12 months (except only for a few days, less than a week, at a time) the possibility of adrenal failure as a result of stress should be borne in mind. (See Medic-Alert, p. 64.)

Breathing exercises, initially administered by the physiotherapist, and subsequently by the mother, may help some children.

Psychological

Excessive parental anxiety and overprotection are frequently important factors in asthmatic children (Berman 1967). Berman described some of the problems of the family background – chronic apprehension, frustration, irritation at the child's illness, sleepless nights (often associated with the child being taken into the parents' bed), parental fatigue, limitation of their activities, expense, and disturbed relationship between the mother and father because of preoccupation with the child's health. Asthma imposes a greater strain on the family than most other illnesses. Some children are kept off school if they have the slightest wheeze – and yet are allowed to go shopping with the mother, to go to the cinema, or to the baby clinic with the new baby. Others are put to bed as soon as they begin to wheeze. As a result of missing school, they become worried about dropping behind, wheeze all the more, and so are kept off school all the longer. This vicious circle must be broken. Asthmatic children should not be kept off school unless it is absolutely essential. Neither is there the slightest point in putting them to bed. They should not be prevented from taking part in sport, if they can manage it, or physical education at school.

Some have described a faulty parent–child relationship long before attacks began (Burton 1968). The family doctor can do a great deal in this matter – much more than a hospital consultant can. Attitudes with which the family doctor must be concerned are excessive parental apprehension and anxiety, not only in the attacks but between the attacks. Parents readily convey their anxiety to the child. They watch him constantly in case he may catch cold, get his feet wet, get overtired, eat this or that imaginary antigen or become overexcited. Parents have been described as 'smothering' their asthmatic children by their overprotection. I have seen severe chronic asthma completely 'cured' by a good child psychiatrist who was able to help the parents with this sort of problem.

Both children and parents are helped by a full explanation of the problem of asthma and of the methods being used to help in their solution. For instance, an older child can be told about respiration and how asthma interferes with it.

Infection

The infective aspect of asthma is mainly relevant as a trigger for an attack, and little can be done to prevent the common upper respiratory tract infections which precipitate attacks. Certainly *the removal of tonsils and adenoids will not help and should never be recommended for the prevention of asthma.* It is just possible that attacks of the so-called 'asthmatic bronchitis' (wheezing in the pre-school child only when he gets a cold) might be aborted by bronchodilators (such as ephedrine) at the beginning of a cold; but I know of no evidence to this effect.

Treatment of the attack

When a child has a bad attack of asthma, it is important to allay his and his parents' anxiety, and to introduce an atmosphere of calm and confidence. A sedative, of which the safest is Chloral, may be useful (0·2–0·5 g. by mouth, depending on the age, or 15 mg./kg./6-hourly). Some have recommended diazepam as a good sedative, but it is not altogether safe for the purpose.

It is important that the child should be given enough fluid. The rapid respirations and perhaps sweating from anxiety may cause dehydration and respiratory acidosis. Maintenance of adequate fluid intake helps in expectoration.

The first drug to use is adrenaline 0·15 ml. of 1 in 1,000 for a small child, and 0·25 ml. for an older one, given subcutaneously. If it has not eased the breathing, I would repeat it in 10–15 minutes, and again in a similar period of time. Pallor, sweating and tachycardia are obvious signs that no more should be given.

So much has been written about the danger of pressurized aerosols that I no longer feel that is is safe to leave them in the hands of patients. There is suggestive evidence that they have been at least partly responsible for the increased death rate from asthma. A fall in the death rate was associated with a reduction in the use of aerosols (Inman & Adelstein 1969). Nevertheless it would be safe for the doctor to administer the dose himself. The danger in abuse of the aerosol by overdosage – some patients using it every half-hour or so throughout the day. It is valuable, however, for parents to have something to treat the child with at night, instead of merely calling in the doctor. If a pressurized aerosol of isoprenaline, or preferably orciprenaline, is used by the parent or the child, with the firm understanding that it must not be used more than three times in the 24 hours, it is safe, a great help and comfort to the parents and child, and saves many nocturnal visits by the family doctor. It must be remembered that pressurized aerosols differ greatly in strength, some containing ten times more isoprenaline than others, and some containing atropine.

Salbutamol (Ventolin) is a recent addition to aerosol treatment (Tattersfield & McNicol 1969). It is safer than the isoprenaline aerosols, and preferable, having less cardiovascular side effects. Given as an aerosol, it is said to be effective for 3–8 hours. It may also be given by mouth as a tablet. Ephedrine may perhaps be of some value in an acute attack, but I doubt it.

The xanthine derivatives are popular but dangerous, and there have been several papers on fatalities resulting from their use. One danger is that the effect tends to be cumulative, and it is essential before prescribing aminophylline or theophylline to determine whether the child has been receiving some other preparations of them hidden under trade names. I saw a child who was receiving daily ten drugs for his asthma; on investigation of the constituents of the various trade preparations I found that he was having four different preparations of isoprenaline and two of aminophylline. He survived. Choline theophyllinate (Choledyl) may provide some relief in mild attacks. It has been said (Rees *et al.* 1967) that aminophylline may relieve airway obstruction but worsen the hypoxaemia. I would advise a family doctor not to administer rectal aminophylline, because the danger is too great and all suppositories are undesirable for psychological reasons. If aminophylline is given, the maximum dose is 3–4 mg./kg.; it should never be given more frequently than 8-hourly; and it must be remembered that ephedrine or allied preparations may potentiate its effect. Any doctor prescribing aminophylline should be fully aware of the side effects (p. 31), should not confuse them with the symptoms of the asthma, and should remember that many fatalities have resulted from its use. I would certainly never give intravenous aminophylline in the home.

An expectorant may help, and potassium iodide may be the most useful (25 mg./kg./day). It must be remembered that prolonged administration of iodides may lead to goitre formation.

Antihistamines are contraindicated in the treatment of asthma, because of their drying effect on the bronchial secretions, which would make the coughing up of mucus more difficult. In the same way cough suppressants are contraindicated.

It is wrong to prescribe antibiotics for every attack of asthma, yet the practice is widespread. It is true that colds often precipitate attacks of asthma, but colds are unaffected by antibiotics. The only place of anti-biotics in the treatment of acute attacks of asthma is the complication of pneumonia or pulmonary collapse. In my opinion any child who is so ill that these complications are suspected should be sent into hospital.

Asthma can be dangerous to life. In hospital other measures are available, such as the use of humidified oxygen, intravenous hydrocortisone, and the correction of dehydration and acidosis by intravenous methods. *A child with a severe attack of asthma which does not respond fairly rapidly to the measures described should be sent to hospital without delay.* There, assisted respiration and bronchoscopic removal of obstructive mucus can save life.

Deaths from asthma are commonly due to the following causes, which are associated with dangerous hypoxia, acidaemic dehydration, cardiac irregularities or combinations of these (Fontana, 1965, Robbins 1966):

overdosage of pressurized aerosols;

overdosage of aminophylline;

bronchial obstruction, often precipitated by the use of xanthine deriva-tives, antihistamines or cough suppressants;

oxygen without humidification;

respiratory acidosis;

oversedation;

corticosteroids;

pneumonia and pulmonary collapse;

heart failure.

Summary

Between attacks

Reduce allergens.

Treat the psychological factor – overprotection; try to allay anxiety in child and parent.

Disodium cromoglycate.

Rarely – corticosteroids for short period.

In attacks

Allay anxiety.

Sedative if necessary.

Attend to fluid balance.

Adrenaline.

Isoprenaline or orciprenaline aerosol.
Salbutamol.
Do not delay transfer to hospital if child is ill and fails to respond.

Preparations referred to

Salbutamol
Tablets Age 3–6 years $\frac{1}{2}$–1 tablet
          6–12 years   1 tablet
          Over 12 years Adult dose
Aerosol

Orciprenaline (Alupent)
20 mg. tablets: $\frac{1}{2}$ tab. q.d. at 6–12 years.

Prednisolone
Trade names include Precortisyl, Prednesol, Prednelan, Deltacortef, Deltacortril etc. I suggest that one prescribes prednisolone.

Tetracosactrin
Trade names synachthen and cortrosyn. Dose 0·25 mg. twice a week. Store below 15°C in the dark.
Dose 0·25 mg. twice a week.

Corticotrophin (ACTH) gelatin BP
Trade name Acthar Gel.

Ephedrine
Age 1 year   7·5 mg. b.d.
Age 7 years 15 mg. b.d.
Puberty   30 mg. b.d.

Choline theophyllinate (Choledyl)
Age 1 year   50 mg. t.d.
Age 7 years 100 mg. t.d.
Puberty   200 mg. t.d.

References

ANON. (1965) Hyposensitisation injections in hay fever and other conditions. *Drug and Therapeutics Bulletin*, **3**, 95.

ANON. (1967) Oral theophyllines – old and new. *Drug and Therapeutics Bulletin*, **5**, 101.

ANON. (1969) Salbutamol for asthma. *Drug and Therapeutics Bulletin*, **7**, 38.

BERMAN S. (1967) The psychological implications of intractable asthma in childhood. *Clinc. Proc. Children's Hospital Dist. Columbia*, **23**, 210.

BURTON L. (1968) *Vulnerable Children*. London, Routledge and Kegan Paul.

FONTANA V.J. (1965) Deaths from asthma in children. *Am. J. Dis. Ch.* **110**, 574.

FONTANA V.J., HOLT L.E. & MAINLAND J.L. (1966) Effectiveness of hyposensitisation therapy in ragweed hay fever in children. *J. Am. Med. Ass.* **195**, 985.

FORGACS P. & SWAN A.V. (1968) Treatment of house dust allergy. *Brit. Med. J.* **3**, 774.

GLASER J. (1969) in Kagan, B.M. & Gellis S.S., *Current Pediatric Therapy*. Chicago, Saunders.

INMAN W.H. & ADELSTEIN A.M. (1969) Rise and fall of asthma mortality in England and Wales in relation to use of pressurised aerosols. *Lancet*, **2**, 279.

JOHNSTONE D.E. & DUTTON A. (1968) The value of hyposensitisation therapy for bronchial asthma in children – a 14 year study. *Pediatrics*, **42**, 793.

MANSMANN H.C. (1968) Management of the child with bronchial asthma. *Ped. Clinics N. America*, **15**, 357.

NOLKE A.C. (1956) Severe toxic effects from aminophylline and theophylline suppositories in children. *J. Am. Med. Ass.* **161**, 693.

PATERSON J.W. (1970) Salbutamol (Ventolin). *Prescribers' Journal*, **10**, 19.

PETERSON R.D.A. (1968) Allergy-status and perspective. *J. Pediat.* **73**, 436, 459.

REES H.A., BORTHWICK R.C., MILLAR J.S. & DONALD K.W. (1967) Aminophylline in bronchial asthma. *Lancet*, **2**, 1167.

ROBBINS J.J. (1966) Asthmatic deaths in children. *J.A.M.A.* **197**, 151.

SOIFER I. (1957) Aminophylline toxicity. *J. Pediat.* **50**, 659.

TATTERSFIELD A.E. & McNICHOL M.W. (1969) Salbutamol and isoproterenol: bronchodilator and cardiovascular activity. *New Engl. J. Med.* **281**, 1323.

ATTENTION-SEEKING DEVICES

These include dirt-eating, pulling the flowers up in the garden, shouting, coughing, turning the gas taps on, swearing and innumerable tricks which the child knows will cause consternation and distress.

Where possible, the trick should be ignored. Punishment will achieve nothing but harm. It is necessary to try to find out why the child feels the need for his behaviour. He may feel that he is not wanted, is not as important as he was (perhaps because of jealousy) or is not loved – perhaps because of excessive strictness, constant scolding, frequent punishment or other unkindness. The family doctor has the difficult task of trying to determine the cause of the child's behaviour. Medicine will not help.

THE BACKWARD CHILD

Hardly any children are exactly average in all aspects of development. Some are later or earlier in beginning to smile, sit, walk, talk, control the bladder, read and pass other milestones. The factors concerned have been discussed in detail in my book, *The Development of the Infant and Young Child: Normal and Abnormal* (Illingworth 1970).

Some children are backward in all aspects of development. The causes of this were also discussed in the above book. The problems of the backward intelligent child were also discussed in my book *The Normal School Child: His Problems Physical and Emotional* (Illingworth 1964). As the causes of backwardness and poor performance in a child in relation to his intelligence are mainly remediable, I have given a brief summary of the causes in the section below, in order that the appropriate treatment can be arranged.

Emotional causes, especially insecurity of any kind, are most important sources of backwardness in relation to intelligence. Hence, any worry at home or school, or anything else which is causing insecurity, must be sought by the family doctor. The help of the school medical officer may be needed. The parents may be advised to discuss the child's problems with his teachers. An educational psychologist may be needed to eliminate specific learning disorders.

Defects of vision and hearing may cause backwardness and pass unrecognized for months or years. Hence these conditions must always be eliminated.

Repeated absences from school, which may be due to the parents' overanxiety or their disregard of the value of education, or to advice, wise or unwise, given by the doctor about keeping the child at home. This is a problem which may occur especially in the case of asthmatic children, or other children who frequently develop colds and coughs. One should constantly question the wisdom of keeping children off school for anything but an acute febrile illness. For instance, it is almost always wrong to quarantine a child because a sibling has some infectious disease – a matter which I have discussed elsewhere (Illingworth 1968).

Antiepileptic drugs, notably phenytoin and phenobarbitone, may lead to backwardness at school – not necessarily in an overdosage. They may cause drowsiness or defective concentration, and phenobarbitone may cause bad behaviour which interferes with school work. If this is suspected, substitute drugs should be tried.

Finally, some parents actively discourage homework, show little interest in the child's education, and provide minimal stimulation to achievement (Illingworth 1968). This is a most difficult situation which it may be impossible to remedy.

References

ILLINGWORTH R.S. (1964) *The Normal School Child: His Problems Physical and Emotional.* London, Heinemann.

ILLINGWORTH R.S. (1968) *The Normal Child.* 4th edn. London, Churchill.

ILLINGWORTH R.S. (1968) How to help a child to achieve his best. *J. Pediat.* 73, 61.

ILLINGWORTH R.S. (1970) *The Development of the Infant and Young Child: Normal and Abnormal.* 4th edn. London, Livingstone.

BALANITIS

Acute balanitis is likely to be a self-righting condition. The foreskin should be retracted and cleaned. Bacitracin ointment may be applied. Pain on passing urine may be reduced if the child passes urine in the bath.

It should not be thought that an attack of balanitis implies that circumcision should be performed; retraction often becomes possible as the result of an attack.

THE BATTERED CHILD ('Child Abuse')

The family doctor is in a key position with regard to the battered child. He may be able to prevent the child being injured, by taking necessary steps. He may well be the first to suspect the diagnosis because of his knowledge of the family background and because he is the first to see the child after his injury; and he is able to help the parents after the child has been treated.

The term 'battered child' is a bad one, in that it does not include several types of injury which the parents may inflict. The term 'child abuse' is preferable. The following are some of the manifestations of child abuse:

bruises;
fractured limbs;
fractured skull;
subdural haematoma;
burns – cigarette burns; electric radiator burns on the buttocks;
poisoning;
laceration of the mouth by forceful insertion of a dummy;
injury to viscera – liver, kidney, spleen performation of intestine;
eye injury;
emotional deprivation and other forms of cruelty;
failure to thrive;
starvation, dehydration.

Poisoning can be achieved by deliberate administration of poison or of an overdose of medicine, or by deliberately leaving poisonous drugs within his reach or giving him a bottle of pills to play with. 'Accidents' can be caused by deliberately allowing a child to fall out of his chair or down the stairs. Kempe estimated that 10 per cent of all casualties under the age of 2, seen at Denver, Colorado, and 25 per cent of all fractures under that age, were inflicted by parents.

The diagnosis is difficult, because child abuse is always denied by the parents. The doctor looks carefully for discrepancies between the history and the physical signs. It is wise to take the history from the mother and father separately, in the absence of the other, in order to look for discrepancies. He becomes suspicious if there has been a notable delay between the stated time of the injury and the time of seeking medical help. He is suspicious if the mother complains that the baby is always crying, or is backward, when he is not. He knows that the common background is one of unhappiness and cruelty in the parents' own childhood. He knows that a mother is worn out and at her wits' end with poverty, frequent child-bearing, a drunken husband and ill health.

When the family doctor suspects child abuse, he should not accuse the parents; he should refer the child to hospital. If he will provide the hospital doctor with a full record of previous episodes, his help in establishing the diagnosis will be invaluable. The difficulty facing the hospital doctor is commonly lack of knowledge of previous episodes; he may not know that the child has previously been sent to another hospital; if there is inadequate co-ordination of notes within his hospital, he may not know, for instance, that the child attending for a fracture was previously treated for burns or other injuries attended to in a different department.

Kempe, who has made important contributions to the study of child abuse, emphasized that the treatment should not consist of punishment of the parents. It certainly does not consist of doing nothing, for that, according to Kempe, is tantamount to signing the child's death warrant; the abuse increases and may well end in the child's death. It consists of giving the parents support, making them feel that someone cares, that they can get help when they feel at their wits' end. The health visitor, the psychiatric social worker and certainly the family doctor, all contribute to the management of the problem.

References

ANON. (1966) The battered baby (middle article). *Brit. Med. J.* 1, 601.

ANON. (1969) Battered babies (leading article). *Brit. Med. J.* 3, 667.

HELFER R.E. & KEMPE C.H. (1968) *The Battered Child.* Chicago, University of Chicago Press.

HELFER R.E. & POLLOCK C.B. (1968) The battered child syndrome. *Advances in Pediatrics*, Vol. XV. New York, Year Book Publishers.

KEMPE C.H. (1971) Paediatric implications of the battered baby syndrome. *Arch. Dis. Childh.* 46, 28.

PICKEL S., ANDERSON C. & HOLLIDAY M.A. (1970) Thirsting and hypernatremic dehydration, a form of child abuse. *Pediatrics*, 45, 54.

BITES

Dog or cat bites are treated in the same way as any other penetrating injury – by cleansing the wound. An antibiotic (*e.g.* penicillin) is prescribed if the wound is dirty, or if suturing has been necessary. In this case a booster dose of tetanus toxoid may be given if the child has not had a dose for three years or more.

BLEPHARITIS

There is commonly an associated scurf of scalp, and this should be treated by daily washing. The blepharitis may be treated by the application of sulphacetamide or bacitracin ointment four times a day, removing any dry scales. Treatment is not altogether satisfactory.

The preparation used is sulphacetamide eye ointment (Albucid) $2\frac{1}{2}\%$, 6%, 10%.

THE BLIND CHILD

The blind child will be under the care of the Local Authority Blind Services, and the parents will be given a great deal of help and advice in his management. The Royal National Institute for the Blind, 224 Great Portland Street, London W1, will also give help and advice. The Local Authority may have a Nursery School and home teachers for blind children.

The family doctor must not feel that he has no part to play in helping the blind child and his family. He can complement the work of the expert bodies which are trying to help the family. A blind child is apt to suffer from 'pseudoretardation' or 'pseudofeeblemindedness' – backwardness resulting from overprotection and deprivation of the normal sensory stimuli which normal children experience. The family doctor can do much to prevent this. Restrictive practices should be reduced to an absolute minimum. It is the natural reaction of the parents of a handicapped child to do everything for him, instead of letting him learn slowly and painfully to do things for himself. The blind child must be allowed to sit, walk, feed himself, attend to his toilet needs, run up and down stairs, climb, splash in a paddling pool, and dance; but while normal children learn spontaneously, the blind child has to be taught. The normal child walks without being taught, but the blind child has to be taught to walk. He must be allowed to feel, squeeze and handle things. He must be given auditory, tactile and oral sensory stimuli. At the appropriate age he should be given a ball to play with, boxes, push and pull toys, bricks, pots and pans and peg boards. For games he can be paired with a child who can see. He can play with dominoes, interlocking bricks, and use Braille letters and card games, writing machines, Braille books, clock and watch. When old enough he may join the scouts and the girl may join the guides. He should be treated as far as possible as a normal child, every effort being made not to regard him as different or to make him feel different.

I have listed three books which deal with the problems of the blind child, that by Spock and Lerrigo being written for parents. Miss Lunt was for eight years a headmistress of a nursery school for blind children administered by the Royal National Institute for the Blind, and her book provides invaluable advice to the parents of blind children.

References

CARNEGIE UNITED KINGDOM TRUST (1964) *Handicapped Children and Their Families.* Dunfermline.
LUNT L. (1965) *If You Make a Noise I Can't See.* London, Gollancz.
SPOCK B. & LERRIGO M.O. (1965) *Caring for your Disabled Child.* London, Macmillan.

BOILS

There is nothing to be gained by giving antibiotics by mouth or injection. They do not shorten the life of a boil or prevent further boils. It is wise, however, to clean the skin around the boil with 50 per cent spirit, hexachlorophane, or chlorhexidine cream BPC three or four times daily, in order to try to prevent further boils. The skin may be washed with hexachlorophane soap. Adhesive tape or other strapping should not be used, because it may irritate the skin and predispose to further infection. If there are recurrent boils, particularly about the face and neck, one should take a swab from the nose, and if staphylococci are cultured, neomycin 0·5 per cent and chlorhexidine 0·1 per cent cream or framycetin cream is applied locally to the nostrils three or four times a day – or other antibiotic depending on the sensitivity of the organism. It must be remembered that antibiotic ointments are liable to sensitize the skin. They are probably justified for local use just in and around the nostril. The urine will be examined for glycosuria.

It is necessary to consider the whole family; there may be a reservoir of infection in another member of the family (*e.g.* chronic antrum infection in the father, or recurrent boils or styes).

When the boil is in an early stage, some recommend the application of dry heat, as from a hot-water bottle, but I am doubtful about the rationale or efficacy of this. A fluctuant boil should be incised.

Finger nails should be kept short, so that scratching does not occur. Every effort should be made to keep the skin scrupulously clean in order to prevent further infection.

The preparations used in treatment are:

hexachlorophane 3% cream (trade preparations: Phisohex, Disfex, Sterzac, Cidal, Gamoflen);

framycetin – trade name Soframycin;

neomycin – chlorhexidine nasal cream (Naseptin);

chlorhexidine – trade name Hibitane.

BOW LEGS

The normal bowing of the legs of the older infant and toddler often causes anxiety. It is almost always a self-righting condition requiring no treatment. It certainly does not require treatment if there is no more than half-an-inch separating the knees when the child is standing with the malleoli touching, and if there is no abnormal weight-bearing, as shown by abnormal shoe wear. Unless the bowing is severe, one should merely observe the child at intervals, only asking for expert advice if deterioration is occurring or if there are grounds for thinking that the child has rickets. If there is doubt, it is better to see the child again in three months in order to remeasure, and then, if necessary, refer the child to an orthopaedic surgeon experienced in children's problems.

In toddlers and young children, marked bowing of the legs may be due to Blount's disease, an acquired disease of unknown aetiology involving the proximal tibial metaphysis and epiphysis; it causes bowing of the legs caused by retardation of the growth of the medial portion of the tibia. It may be treated by a brace and occasionally by osteotomy. The condition has to be distinguished from severe rickets by X-ray and biochemical investigation. There are other and rarer conditions associated with bowing of the legs, and these demand expert orthopaedic treatment.

BREATH-HOLDING ATTACKS

See *Convulsions*, p. 126.

Breath-holding attacks occur when the child is hurt, frightened or thwarted. It is a mistake to regard all breath-holding attacks as a behaviour problem or to treat them as such. The type of attack which occurs when the child is hurt is similar to a faint or vasovagal attack in an adult, and is in no way related to mismanagement by the mother. If the attack occurs only when he is thwarted, it is important that as little fuss as possible should be made, and that on no account should he have his own way as a result of the attack. He may be caused to take a breath by pinching his ear, holding him upside down or dashing cold water over his face.

Antiepileptic drugs have no place in the management of this condition. It will resolve by the age of 5 or 6, and often sooner; but despite all one's efforts, the attacks may commonly continue until that age.

It is by no means always easy to distinguish breath-holding attacks from epilepsy. If the family doctor is doubtful about the diagnosis, the advice of a paediatrician should be sought; he too may find it difficult to be sure of the diagnosis. It would certainly be undesirable to administer antiepileptic drugs unnecessarily, because of their many side effects; and it is better to try to reach a definite diagnosis of breath-holding attacks, so that the mother's anxiety can be allayed.

BRONCHIECTASIS

A child with bronchiectasis will be under the surveillance of a consultant. The treatment depends on the cause. It will include treatment of the associated antrum infection by antibiotics and possibly antral washouts; the child will be given postural drainage and probably antibiotics in an attempt to eradicate the organisms to which they have been shown to be sensitive. Surgical treatment may be advised if the condition is localized, but this is an uncommon procedure in childhood.

The family doctor will prescribe intensive antibiotic therapy for acute exacerbatious and superadded respiratory infections. He may be asked to see that the child is given postural drainage. This should not be haphazard. It is the responsibility of the radiologist to determine which bronchus or bronchi are involved, because the position for postural drainage depends on this. For instance, the upper lobe bronchus drains best when the child is up and about. For the remaining bronchi, the child sleeps in the appropriate position. For the middle, ventral, and anterior basal bronchus the child sleeps on his back, with a wedge under the affected side, with the foot of the bed raised 18–24 in. The feet must be fixed. For the axillary basal, posterior basal and dorsal bronchi the child sleeps prone, tilted, with the chest and head down (*e.g.* with a mattress rolled up in the centre of the bed and another on top of it) and with a wedge under the affected side.

BRONCHIOLITIS

It is wise to send most infants with bronchiolitis into hospital, where it is easier to give adequate treatment in the way of oxygen and a humidified atmosphere, than it is in the home. It is extremely difficult, if not impossible, to distinguish clinically severe acute bronchiolitis from bronchopneumonia, and radiological examination is likely to be necessary to make the distinction. The treatment of the two conditions is different, for acute bronchiolitis is usually due to the respiratory syncitial virus which is not sensitive to antibiotics (though some cases are due to staphylococci or pneumococci) while bronchopneumonia usually responds to penicillin and other drugs.

The Newcastle workers (Holdaway *et al.* 1967), after a detailed study of a large number of infants with acute bronchiolitis, concluded that it was much more important to correct the dehydration, secondary hypoxia and heart failure, than to give antibiotics. They recommended that benzyl penicillin together with cloxacillin should be given until the results of radiological, virological and bacteriological investigations were available; the antibiotics should then be discontinued if there is no evidence of consolidation, and if staphylococcus aureus or haemophilus influenzae are not cultured from the cough swab. They recommended hydration, the administration of oxygen, digoxin if necessary, amylobarbitone as a sedative (15–30 mg. 6-hourly), but no antibiotic, corticosteroid or bronchodilator drugs.

Various workers suggested that corticosteroids were of value in this condition, but subsequent carefully controlled work (Connolly *et al.* 1969) showed that they are useless.

Several experts have emphasized the important of adequate hydration in these children. Humidification is also a help.

Expert nursing is essential, and I strongly advocate that children with acute bronchiolitis should be sent to a Children's Hospital or Children's Unit.

References

CONNOLLY J.H., FIELD C.M.B., GLASGOW J.F.T., SLATTERY C.M. & MACLYNN D.M. (1969) A double blind trial of prednisolone in epidemic bronchiolitis due to respiratory syncytial virus. *Acta Paediat. Scandinavica*, 58, 116.

HOLDAWAY D., ROMER A.C. & GARDNER P.S. (1967) The diagnosis and management of bronchiolitis. *Pediatrics*, 39, 924.

BRUISE UNDER FINGER NAIL: TRAPPED FINGER

The temptation to remove the finger nail must always be resisted. No treatment is required unless there is tension under the nail, causing pain, in which case the end of a paper clip is made red-hot and the nail is trephined by it to relieve the pressure. Otherwise if the nail is left alone it may separate spontaneously in a few weeks, in which case a new nail will be found under it.

THE BULLIED CHILD

It is not easy to define precisely the causes of bullying. The main cause is probably the child's timid personality and his inability or unwillingness to stand up for himself. His personality, as always, is partly inherited and partly the result of his environment.

The family doctor has two alternatives when his advice is sought about a child's symptoms when they are due to bullying. He can get in touch with the headmaster (or school medical officer); or he can recommend steps which will give the child self-confidence and enable him to deal effectively with a bully. I suggest that Judo or similar classes be arranged for the child. It is better for the child to find his own answer to the problem than to have the matter dealt with by the school.

BURNS

For any but a trivial burn, the child is sent to hospital immediately.

As an immediate first-aid measure, it is suggested that the burnt limb should be immersed for a few minutes in iced water, if it is available. If it is a small burn, the affected area and the skin around are cleaned with 1 per cent cetrimide, a clean dry dressing is applied and the burnt area is sealed off completely with an adhesive dressing, *e.g.* 'Surgifix' tubular bandage. It is then left undisturbed for a week – but is not allowed to get wet. Tulle gras or Viocutin (Tulle with silver nitrate) is a convenient safe covering. Blisters should *not* be incised unless they are very tense and painful, or spread over the crease of a joint, such as that of a finger, in which case they are pricked by a sterile needle; they provide a safe protective cover if left intact. Again, the dressing should be left intact for a week. The removal of a dressing is painful, predisposes to infection, and pulls off a healing area. Antibiotics are not used as a routine. If a sedative is used for the first night, paracetamol may be prescribed.

When a more severely burnt child comes home from hospital, the family doctor may have to deal with the psychological problems resulting from the burn and the stay in hospital. The mother may feel guilt because of the fact of the burn; the child, on return home after painful experiences in hospital, may be aggressive and anxious, or may develop other behaviour problems. The child should not be spoilt, but should be given normal loving discipline without favouritism at the cost of his siblings.

If there is any indication that a contracture is beginning to develop in a burnt area, the child should be referred back to hospital for advice.

References

SNEDDON J. (1964) The treatment of burns in the casualty department. *Practitioner*, 193, 768.
WOODWARD J.M. (1968) The burnt child and his family. *Proc. Roy. Soc. Med.* 61, 1087.

CATARRH

See *Antrum Infection*, *Allergic Rhinitis*, *Colds* and *Adenoids*.

CEPHALHAEMATOMA

A cephalhaematoma in a newborn baby must be left alone. It is always wrong to aspirate it, because of the risk of introducing an infection.

CEREBRAL PALSY

A child with suspected or confidently diagnosed cerebral palsy should be referred to a paediatrician, who will assess the child and arrange for specialist treatment. The child needs treatment to learn independence in sitting, walking, talking, dressing and feeding himself and attending to his toilet needs – and an expert physiotherapist, speech therapist and occupational therapist will be needed; he will have his hearing tested because of the frequency of deafness, and his eyesight tested, because of the frequency of visual defects; he will have his intelligence assessed, so that guidance can be given on the choice of school; and deformities must be prevented, so that toe walking does not develop, and the hip does not become dislocated by the pull of spastic muscles.

The parents must play their part in the treatment of the child, and the family doctor can do much to help them. He has to counsel the mother on management and outlook, and with regard to her own feelings about the child. He has to help the parents not to show favouritism to the child at the cost of the siblings, nor to overprotect the child and prevent him from learning to look after himself. The doctor has to enable the child to make the most of the use of his limbs, to come to terms with his handicap, to avoid resentment, loneliness and isolation. Parents do not often show rejection of a handicapped child, but, if they do, the family doctor can help the parents to overcome any such rejection. They are more likely to show a pathological attachment to the child, at the cost of the normal siblings, allowing the whole home to revolve around the handicapped child. The family doctor may try to find ways in which the child can make himself useful and do things to help his mother. The family doctor can guide the parents with regard to giving the child the essential sensory stimuli – visual, auditory and tactile – which otherwise the child would miss and so unnecessary retardation might result. He can give them guidance about joining a parents' association, and as to the child's education, play and learning.

Medicines play practically no part in the treatment of cerebral palsy. So-called muscle-relaxants (*e.g.* Carisoprodol 'Soma') have proved to be without value in the management of these children. It is possible that chlorpromazine or chlordiazepoxide may help a little with regard to the spasticity, but the evidence for this is uncertain.

In the spastic form of cerebral palsy there is a danger of obesity, especially around puberty, as a result of inactivity. This must be prevented, because if the child cannot walk, it greatly adds to the mother's difficulties.

For the treatment of epileptic fits in spastic children, see *Epilepsy* (p. 160).

Parents should be encouraged to join the local branch of the Spastic Society. The central address is The Spastics Society, 12 Park Crescent, London w1.

References

CARDWELL V.E. (1947) *The Cerebral Palsied Child and his Care in the Home.* New York, Association for the Aid of Crippled Children.

GIRARD P.M. (1937) *The Home Treatment of Spastic Paralysis.* Philadelphia, Lippincott.

SHERIDAN MARY D. (1965) *The Handicapped Child and his Home.* Harpenden, National Children's Home.

SPOCK B. & LERRIGO M.O. (1965) *Caring for your Disabled Child.* New York, Macmillan.

CHALAZION

This is a cyst on the lid margin due to obstruction of a meibomian gland. It is treated by excision, but if it has become infected an antibiotic ointment such as sulphacetamide or neomycin may be applied until the infection has settled down. If the chalazion is a large infected one, initial incision may be required, prior to excision.

CHICKENPOX

No medicine or lotion is normally required for the child with chickenpox. The child is kept off school but not in bed. Scarring is the result of scratching and infecting the vesicles. His finger nails should be kept short and clean so that damage done by scratching is minimized. He should be discouraged from scratching, and if itching is serious, chlorpheniramine (Piriton) 0·35 mg./kg./day may be prescribed in four divided doses; but it is doubtful whether it is really necessary. Calamine lotion may help to reduce the itching. Hexachlorophane soap may help to prevent infection. *Normally no medical treatment of any kind is required, but the skin should be kept clean and the nails clean and short.*

Duration of infectivity – 1 day before the rash appears to 6 days after its appearance. Quarantine is not required.

Incubation period: 15–18 days.

CHILBLAINS

There is no indication for drug treatment of chilblains. Calcium preparations and calciferol are useless, and the latter is dangerous; their use was irrational. Nicotinic acid is ineffective. Phenoxybenzamine has been tried, but side effects are troublesome in 25–30 per cent.

The only profitable measure to prevent chilblains is to keep the hands and feet warm. It is said that the hands and feet should be warmed by exercise rather than by local heat (in front of a fire, etc.). As far as possible, extreme changes of temperature should be avoided.

Reference

ANON. (1965) Treatment for Chilblains. *Drug and Therapeutics Bulletin*, **3**, 90.

CHOANAL ATRESIA

When a baby at birth becomes severely cyanosed and cannot breathe when his mouth is shut, he is likely to have choanal atresia, a web at the back of the nose. Babies do not open the mouth to breathe if the nose is obstructed until about 4 months of age, and choanel atresia causes severe respiratory distress as soon as the baby is born. As soon as he opens his mouth to cry, the colour returns to normal.

The immediate treatment is to insert an airway into the mouth. As soon as this is done the child breathes normally. There is then no urgency about the situation. The baby is taken to hospital and in the next two or three days the ear, nose and throat surgeon will carry out an elective operation.

CHOREA

Chorea is rarely seen now and severe cases in this country are now extremely rare. Unless the family doctor can estimate the erythrocyte sedimentation rate (ESR) and find it normal, or if there is a cardiac murmur, the child should be referred to hospital for treatment; but if the ESR and the heart are normal, and the chorea is only mild, the child could well be treated at home. The child should be kept off school. Although it has been customary to prescribe phenobarbitone, I doubt whether it is necessary. I would not think that rest in bed is necessary. If the diagnosis is correct, the chorea should subside within six weeks at the most.

A psychological upset may precipitate an attack of chorea, and hence possible emotional factors should be looked for and treated. The common mistake is to confuse tics or overactivity with chorea.

CIRCUMCISION

The whole question of circumcision has been discussed by me elsewhere (Illingworth 1968). The operation is largely a needless ritual, which is unpleasant for the child. Morgan (1967) wrote: 'The American public has come to view circumcision in the same light as the other essentials of life, namely superhighways, refrigerators and television sets. As well deprive these citizens of their birthright as suggest that they retain their prepuce. It has become imperative to lop it off to keep up with the Jones, for in the affluent society, status and a foreskin are incompatible.' Bolande (1969) likens circumcision to other rituals, such as the extraction or knocking out of teeth, practised as a manhood initiation rite, a female pubertal rite or a propitiatory sacrifice. Other similar operations are uvulectomy, infibulation in the girl, and castration.

Øster (1968) pointed out that it is incorrect to use the term 'adhesions' for the common epithelium separating the inner surface of the prepuce and the glans. Separation results from keratinization of the cells under the influence of androgens, and occurs as a normal biological process in school life. In a study of Copenhagen schoolboys aged 6–17 years, with 9,545 observations, he found that the foreskin had not retracted in 8 per cent at the age of 6–7 years, but had not retracted in only 1 per cent at the age of 16–17 years.

Briefly, the only firm medical indication for circumcision is such severe scarring of the foreskin due to neglected ammonia dermatitis that retraction is and will be impossible. Severe balanitis with pus formation might be another indication when the infection has subsided if the foreskin cannot be retracted. Circumcision is *never* to be advised simply because the mother, father, aunt or mother-in-law wants it done. The child alone matters, and the operation should never be carried out unless it is necessary for him.

It is nonsense to perform a circumcision because the foreskin is a long one ('Redundant foreskin'): because of a so-called pinhole meatus – a non-existent condition; because the foreskin balloons when the boy passes urine (it always does, if the foreskin happens to lie over the meatus at the time of micturition); or because the foreskin cannot be retracted (it can, unless there has been neglected ammonia dermatitis; but no effort should be made to do so until the child is at least 3 or 4). It should not be done to prevent syphilis (there are other ways of preventing that infection), or to prevent carcinoma of the penis or cervix (another myth).

Complications of the operation include death (16–20 per year in England and Wales), psychological trauma (if the operation is done without an anaesthetic, as it is in some countries), haemorrhage, sepsis, gangrene of the penis, mutilation of the penis, obstruction by removal of too little mucosa, urinary fistula (as a result of passing a needle through the urethra when stitching a bleeding point), and hiding the corona (as a result of sewing the skin edge to the glans). If the operation is done at a time when there is ammonia dermatitis, a meatal ulcer may develop.

References

BOLANDE R.P. (1969) Ritualistic surgery – Circumcision and tonsillectomy. *New Engl. J. Med.* **280**, 591.
GAIRDNER D. (1949) The fate of the foreskin. *Brit. Med. J.* **2**, 1433.
ILLINGWORTH R.S. (1968) *The Normal Child.* London, Churchill.
MORGAN W.K.C. (1967) Penile plunder. *Australian Med. J.* **1**, 1102.
ØSTER J. (1968) Further fate of the foreskin. *Arch. Dis. Childh.* **43**, 200.
PRESTON E.N. (1970) Whither the foreskin? *J. Am. Med. Ass.* **213**, 1853.

CLEFT PALATE

A cleft palate presents obvious feeding difficulties, and an acrylic prosthesis is inserted a few days after birth. The cleft palate itself will be closed between 12 and 18 months of age. Tonsils must not be removed because of the effect of scarring, and adenoids must not be removed because the removal of the pad of adenoids prevents the short palate from closing off the oropharynx.

Until the prosthesis can be fitted, the baby may be fed by pipette or spoon.

E

Orthodontic treatment and speech therapy may be required after repair of the palate.

THE CLUMSY CHILD

The numerous causes of clumsiness in children have been discussed in my book *Common Symptoms of Disease in Children* (Illingworth 1971). Unless the clumsiness is due to a drug (*e.g.* antiepileptic), or to emotional factors, there is no cause for which specific treatment is possible. It is vitally important, however, that the teachers should know that the child's bad writing and other signs of clumsiness are not due to naughtiness. Teachers who realize that the child cannot help being clumsy will be kind and sympathetic; if they think that the child is just naughty, they make him worse by unkindness in an attempt to cure him by discipline. Hence the family doctor should be ready to contact the head teacher (or better still, the School Medical Officer), so that the child's problems are better understood. Physiotherapy is not of value for this condition.

The causes of clumsiness are numerous and complex, and I would advise the family doctor to refer an affected child to a paediatrician for full neurological assessment, if necessary with the help of a child psychologist – for some of these children have severe defects of spatial appreciation.

COELIAC DISEASE

A child with suspected coeliac disease will be referred to a paediatrician for establishment of the diagnosis. This is essential before treatment can be given, for even if the presence of steatorrhoea is confirmed, there are many other causes of steatorrhoea, and coeliac disease is not the most common (the commonest being fibrocystic disease of the pancreas). Once a gluten-free diet has been started, it is much less easy to establish the diagnosis, and a long delay in establishing it is almost inevitable.

The paediatrician will almost certainly admit the child in order to start him on a gluten-free diet, and discharge him to the care of the family doctor when weight gain is satisfactory. He will supply a diet sheet, but for the guidance of the family doctor I have printed below instructions modified from the book, *Diets for Sick Children* by Francis, D.E.M. and Dixon, D.J.W. Oxford, Blackwell Scientific Publications. It should be noted that occasionally changes are made in the constituents of proprietary foods, so that a food which is initially gluten-free may later become unsuitable because gluten has been included in it. As far as we know, the dietary details below are accurate.

GLUTEN FREE DIET SHEET
FOODS ALLOWED

Milk – fresh, tinned, powdered.
Meat – fish, fresh or frozen.
Eggs.
Cheese, cream cheese.
Fruit – tinned, fresh, cooked, dried.
Vegetables – fresh, cooked, frozen, dried.
Maize or corn.
Soya, barley, oats, rice, tapioca, sago.
Pure wheat starch.
Rite Diet gluten free flour.
Prepared cereals made from above.
Robinsons Baby Rice or Groats.
Cornflakes.
Rice Krispies.
Gluten free bread, pastry, cakes, biscuits, puddings from rice oats and/or corn or soya flour, wheat starch or Rite Diet gluten free flour.
Soups, sauces and gravy made with meat, vegetables and thickened with cornflour, barley, sago, rice, wheat starch, Bisto, Bovril, *bottled* Oxo.
Sugar, honey, jam, marmalade, plain boiled sweets or lollies, plain chocolate.
Butter, margarine, oil, cream.
Animal fats (all must be used in moderation only).
Salt, pepper, pure herbs.
Spices and curry.
Tea, coffee, instant coffee,
Squash, fizzy drinks.
Gelatine, rennet, Marmite, Bovril.
See Manufactured products also.

FOODS FORBIDDEN

Sausages containing bread.
Mince or tinned foods containing flour.
Ham or bacon cooked in bread crumbs.
Cheese spreads containing flour.
Fruit pies or flans.

Vegetable dishes containing wheat, rye or flour.
Wheat or rye or anything containing these.
Semolina, pastas, macaroni, spaghetti, noodles.
Weetabix, Puffed wheat, grapenuts.
Bemax, Farleys Rice Cereal, Trufoods Junior Cereal.
All bread, biscuits, pastry, cakes made from wheat or rye flour including crispbreads, starch-reduced rolls and slimming products.
Soups, sauces and gravies containing wheat or rye flour, noodles, etc.
Oxo cubes.
Liquorice, ice-cream, sweets, unless listed as gluten free.
Bengers, Ovaltine, Horlicks, chocolate beverages.

GLUTEN FREE MANUFACTURED PRODUCTS

Baby foods

GERBER
Strained

Chicken broth	Beef dinner	Veg. with liver and bacon
Apple	Apricots and orange	Banana and pineapple
Egg custard and rice	Fruit dessert	Orange pudding
Pears and pineapple	Pears	

Junior

Beef dinner	Vegetable and chicken
Pineapple and apricot	Apricots and orange
Fruit dessert	Peaches
Bananas and pineapple	Pears and pineapple
Pears	

HEINZ
Strained

Beef dinner	Beef broth
Bone and veg. broth	Chicken soup
Carrots	Vegetable and lamb broth
Raspberry and apple and rosehip dessert	Apples
Apricot and rice	Apricot custard
Egg custard and rice	Banana dessert
Tomato soup	Fruit dessert
Orange and rosehip dessert	Orange pudding
Peaches	Orange and apricot dessert
Pineapple and rice	Pears
	Creamed cereal

J. & J. COLMAN – ROBINSONS
Baby syrups
Instant Foods
Vegetable and chicken
Rice and hazelnuts

TRUFOODS

Spoonfoods

Buttered carrots	Orange delight and Vit. C.
Pineapple and rice with Vit. C.	Apples, rosehip syrup and Vit. C.
Fruit delight and Vit. C.	Grape jelly
Banana and blackcurrant pudding with Vit. C	

Junior

Apricot treat	Cherry treat
Pineapple delight	Apples in blackcurrant sauce with Vit. C
Fruit and rice with cherries	
Sweetlime dessert with Vit. C	Bananas, blackcurrant and cereal with Vit. C
Fruit in honey sauce with Vit. C	

CEREALS

Baby

Cow & Gate Cereal Food

Farleys gluten free rusks

Heinz Nil

Liga gluten free biscuits

J. & J. Colman (Robinsons) Baby Rice, Groats ready cooked, Barley cereal, Sweet corn, Patent Barley, Patent Groats

Scotts Twin Pack *Oats* only

Trufood Baby Cereal

Breakfast

Allinsons Windmill Oat Flakes

Kellogg Co Ltd Cornflakes, Sugar Stars, Frosties, Rice Crispies, Coco Krispies, Sugar Ricicles

Lyons Ready Brek

Quaker Oat Crunchies, Quick Quaker Oats

Scotts Flying Start, M.O.F., Porage Oats, Ready cooked Groats

BREAD, BISCUITS, CAKES

Welfare Foods Ltd Ripe Diet gluten free bread; Rite Diet biscuits; plain, sweet and chocolate coated rusks; tinned Ripe Diet protein free bread with salt

Lyons Meringues

Davy & Styans gluten free bread and biscuits

FLOURS

Energen Wheat starch

Rakusen Farina Potato Flour

Procea Ltd (Dublin) Titamyl gluten free flour

Welfare Foods Ltd Ripe Diet gluten free flour with or without yeast

Brown & Polson Ltd Patent cornflour

Boots Besyet cornflour

Greens Cornflour

PASTAS
Carlo Orba (U.K.) Ltd Aprosen Macaroni (Rigatini), Aprosen Ringlets (Anelleni), Aprosen Noodles (Tagliatelle)

DRINKS
Beechams All fruit drinks and Lucozade
Birds Maxwell House Coffee
Britanol Ltd Calfresh
Cadburys Drinking Chocolate, Bournvita, Bournville cocoa, Marvel
Carnation Milk – evaporated, coffee mate, Instant Breakfast Food
Frys Cocoa
Glaxo Complan, Casilan
Greens Lemonade powder
Lyons Bev, Chico, Instant coffee
Nestlés Nescafé, Ricory, Nestea, Milo, Nesquick – all flavours, All milks
Rayners Ltd Crusha Milk Shake syrup
Robinsons Soft drinks and squashes
Rowntrees Cocoa powder
Trufood All milk products and substitutes
Unigate, Cow & Gate, Regal All milks

SANDWICH SPREADS, ETC
Bovril Ltd Bovril, Marmite
Gales Honey – all types, lemon curd, lemon cheese, peanut butter – smooth, crunchy
Frys Chocolate spread
Fowlers golden syrup, golden syrup jelly, treacle
Heinz Sandwich spread
Kraft Liquid honey, chutneyed honey
Brands Salmon spread, Crab spread, Potted beef with butter, Calf's foot jelly.

CHEESE SPREAD AND PROCESSED CHEESES
Kraft (Processed Cheeses) Processed cheese (5 lb. loaf), De Luxe Cheddar slices, Old English slices, Cheddar cheese portions, De Luxe Cheshire slices, Dairylea slices, Gruyère cheese portions, Old English cheese spread
Kraft (Cheese spreads) Dairylea cheese spread, Cheese spread with onion, Cheese spread with shrimp, Relli cheese spread, Stardale cheese spread, Blue cheese spread with ham, Velveeta cheese foods, Cheese spread with tomato, Cheese spread with mushroom, Cheese spread with butter, Cheez Whiz, Variety pack cheeses
Nestlés Swiss Knight – Processed Gruyère – Cheese spread – Sandwich slices

MEATS AND PREPARED DISHES
Birds Eye (Frozen) Plaice fillets, Cod fillets, Haddock fillets, Buttered kippers, Buttered smoked kippers, Haddock steaks, Cod steaks, Chicken quarters, Chicken joints
Chef Herrings in tomato sauce
Crosse & Blackwell Herrings in tomato, Kippers, Beans and beef curry

DESSERTS, CUSTARDS AND PUDDINGS

Ambrosia Cream, Creamed Rice, Sago, Tapioca

Brown & Polson Custard powder – all varieties

Birds Eye Mousse, raspberries, strawberries

Cow & Gate Creamed Ground Rice, Tapioca, Sago.

Green's Carmelle, custard powder, Complete custard mix, Blancmange powder, Chocolate blancmange powder, Jelly crystals

Rowntrees Table jellies

Birds Custard powder, blancmange powder, Instant Whip, Jelly de luxe, Lemon pie filling, Dream Topping, Angel Delight.

Boots Custard powder

Carltona Custard powder, jellies

Dietade Dessert moulds

Lyons Mousse

Heinz Mincemeat

Little Miss Muffet Rennet

Morton Pie fillings

Ski Yoghurts

SWEETS

Bassets Jelly babies, Jelly beans, Dolly mixtures, Wine gums, Mixed fruits

Cadburys Block chocolate, chocolate covered assortments, Milk Chocolate, Fruit and Nut, Bournville chocolate Fruit and Nut

Callard & Bowser All lines

Clarnico Peppermint creams, Chocolate mint creams, Pancho chocolate raisins, Pancho chocolate peanuts, Dairy fudge, Fruit jellies.

Frys 5-centre creams, Assorted creams, Chocolate cream, Peppermint cream, Double milk sandwich block, Sandwich block, Crunchie, Chocolate bar, 5-boys milk chocolate, Crunch block

Fuller Kunzle Mint meringue

Keiller Boiled sweets

Mars Limited Opal fruits and mints, Galaxy, Glees, Spangles, Topic, Tunes

Nestlés All chocolate bars

Pascall James Barley sugar squares, Blackcurrant eclairs, Butterscotch, Butter brazils, Court fruit drops, Eclairs, Fruit bonbons, Mint chews, Mitchem mints, Murray candy mints, Murray clear mints, Murray mints and super mints, Murray fruits and super fruits, Fruit chews, Fruit salad, Glucose fruits, Golden barley sugar, Golden barley mints, White Heather assortment.

Lyons Cornish dairy brick, Kup, Choc ice, Orange Maid, King choc, King sundae, Cornish Mivvi, Koola Kreema, Koola Fruta, Sea Jet (not vanilla), standard bars, Mint Hit, Zoom, Fab, giant bars, Cornish bars, Family vanilla brick, Apple and blackberry dessert brick, Cassata dessert brick, Strawberry ripple dessert brick, Fruit caprice dessert brick

George Payne All products

Rowntrees Aeromilk, Aero plain and milk, Aero peppermint, After Eight thin mints, After Eight dessert chocolate, Fruit pastilles, Fruit gums, Jelly tots, Polo mints, Polo fruits, Beechnut chewing gum

Terrys Bitter chocolate, Plain dessert chocolate, Chocolate burnt almonds

Tobler – Meltis Toblerone, New Berry Fruits, twin pack milk and plain Ballerina assortment, Symphony assortment, Chocolate brazils, Chocolate caramels – milk and plain, Chocolate ginger, Tina

Fudge – vanilla and assorted, Orchard Fruits, Fruit pastilles, Crystallized ginger, Orange and lemon slices, Pekin figs, Assorted chocolate liqueurs, Cherries in brandy, Raisins in rum, Après Ski, Crème de menthe liqueurs, Easter eggs, Tobler filled bars – vodka and lime, cherry brandy

Walls Ice lollies – Lemonade Snowfrute, Chocolate Snowe, Woppa orange, Woppa lemon, Woppa raspberry orange, Woppa Choc Tok, Woppa chocolate banana, Orange Sparkle, Sky Ray, Wiz, Hearts.

All standard ice-cream without biscuit, all dairy ice-cream without biscuit including non-milk fat ice-creams, Vanilla brickette, Gaytime tubs, Golden vanilla choc bar,

Popular sweets: Vanilla, Strawberry Fayre, Raspberry Ripple

Family sweets Vanilla, Neapolitan, Raspberry Ripple, Chocolate Carnival, Pineapple Royale, Strawberry Fayre, Orange Galore, Harlequin.

Cornish Ice Cream: Catering shapes, Brickettes, Family sweet, Strawberry Splice

Wilkinsons Jelly babies, Dolly mixtures, Mint imperials

Wrigleys Chewing gums – Juicy Fruit, Double Mint, Arrowmint, P.K. Spearmint

SAUCES, SPICES AND GRAVIES

Bovril Limited Bovril, Marmite, Virol

Brands Beef essence, Chicken essence

Cerebos Bisto, Salt, Pepper

Chef Chef sauce, Tomato ketchup

Crosse & Blackwell Branston pickle, Branston sauce, French capers, Gherkins, Mixed pickle, Olives, Onions pickled, Sweet mixed pickle, Tomato ketchup, Walnuts, Salad cream, Vinegar, Malt and distilled

H.P. Tomato ketchup, Mint sauce, Vinegar

Lea and Perrins Salad cream

Oxo Lemco beef stock tablets, Lemco chicken stock tablets, Oxo beef drink, Bifti

Heinz Salad cream, Mayonnaise, Tomato ketchup, Ideal sauce, Worcestershire sauce, Indian mango chutney, Stem ginger, Malt vinegar, Distilled vinegar, Ideal pickle, Pickled gherkins, all Pickled onions, Pickled walnuts, Mixed pickles, Olives, Olive oil, Piccalilli, Gravy browning, Curry powder, Herbs

Kraft Salad cream, Tomato chutney, Catalina dressing, Miracle French dressing, Barbecue sauce, Roka blue cheese dressing, Tomato ketchup, Coleslaw dressing, French dressing, Oil and vinegar dressing, 1000 Island dressing, Casino dressing

SOUPS

Crosse & Blackwell Cream of tomato, Hawaiian tomato, Real turtle

Heinz Ready to serve: Beef broth, Chicken broth with rice, Cream of green pea, Cream of tomato, Scottish vegetable with lentils; Condensed: Beef broth, Cream of tomato, French style onion, Scotch broth, Tomato soup with rice.

VEGETABLES

Cadburys Smash

Crosse & Blackwell Baked beans, Peas – processed marrowfat

Findus Potato puffles

Heinz Baked beans in tomato sauce, Baked beans in pork flavoured sauce, Curried
    beans, Potato salad, Vegetable salad
Morton Canned vegetables
Smedleys Tinned and frozen vegetables
Smiths Crisps

There has been a difference of opinion as to how long the diet should
continue. There is a risk that if gluten is introduced during childhood, the
child's growth in height may be slowed, or else he may again develop
symptoms of coeliac disease. Once a child has had a normal diet, it may
be difficult to get him to revert to a strict gluten-free diet. Furthermore,
if gluten-containing foods are allowed, the patient is apt to develop folate
deficient anaemia in adolescence. There is a more serious danger, the
development of malignant changes in the intestine, and for this reason
alone it is thought to be the correct treatment to continue the gluten-free
diet indefinitely.

Supportive treatment includes Vitamin D and iron for anaemia.

It is not uncommon to find that after a time a child with coeliac disease
becomes less well than he was and fails to gain weight. The usual explanation of this is that someone (the parent or granny) is giving the child
forbidden foods. The family doctor may be able to discover the facts and
remedy the situation.

The parents should be encouraged to join the Coeliac Society,
P.O. Box 181, London NW2. The society issues an excellent booklet with
diet lists.

COLD INJURY

It would be wise to refer a baby with cold injury or severe hypothermia to
hospital for treatment. The causes are exposure to cold, a response to a
severe infection and, rarely, hypothydroidism.

The treatment is to rewarm slowly over a period of 24–48 hours in a
room having a temperature of about 70°F (19°C). *The temptation to warm the
baby rapidly must be firmly resisted, for it greatly increases the risk of
hypoglycaemia and death.* Only if the hypothermia is extreme, below 30°C,
can rapid rewarming be considered, and that must be done in hospital.

It is probably wise to cover the treatment with an antibiotic such as
kanamycin in case there is an infection, and to ensure adequate fluid
intake.

COLDS (Coryza)

No treatment is needed for the common cold. It is a self-limiting disease caused by a variety of viruses and is unaffected by medicines. There is no need to prescribe drops for the baby's nose. They are apt to have a secondary congestant action and it is said that they may damage the cilia. Oily nose drops should on no account be used because of the danger that they will enter the lung and cause lipoid pneumonia.

There is no justification at all for prescribing an antibiotic for a cold, for the viruses responsible for colds are unaffected by antibiotics. Antibiotics must not be expected to prevent the common complications or sequelae of a cold, such as tracheitis or bronchitis.

The troublesome postnasal discharge after the acute stage is discussed under the section entitled *Cough*. Apart from causing the child to sleep in the prone position, no treatment is available. If a definite antrum infection follows the cold, this should be treated (see *Antrum Infection*). The same applies to the common complication, otitis media, which demands prompt antibiotic therapy.

COLIC, EVENING ('Three Months Colic')

By evening colic ('three months colic') I mean rhythmical screaming attacks in well thriving babies in the evenings of the first two or three months. In the case of breast-fed babies it is important to distinguish it from milk shortage, for there is commonly some deficiency of milk in the evenings, whereas during the day the mother produces sufficient for the baby's needs. It must also be distinguished from crying for company or crying from boredom. If the crying stops when the baby is picked up, it is not what I term 'Evening colic'.

If the diagnosis is correct it responds to dicyclomine hydrochloride (Merbentyl), a teaspoonful of the syrup before the evening feed.

The condition is self-limiting, ceasing by three or possibly (in severe cases) four months.

COLON, IRRITABLE

See *Diarrhoea.*

CONCUSSION

The child with concussion, however brief the unconsciousness, will be referred to the hospital for X-ray of skull and observation. He is likely to be kept in hospital for 24–48 hours and watched carefully for signs of an extradural haemorrhage. The child with an uncomplicated fracture of the skull will probably be detained for about five days.

Normal exercise and activity is allowed on return home.

CONJUNCTIVITIS

In my baby clinic, when I see a baby with conjunctivitis, I take a conjunctival swab for culture and sensitivity studies, and treat with a broad spectrum antibiotic, such as neomycin drops ($\frac{1}{2}$ per cent). If the response is not satisfactory, I then refer to the bacteriological report and alter the treatment accordingly. The possibility of a gonococcal conjunctivitis must be remembered. Before instilling the drops, the mother should wipe away pus with moistened cotton wool.

After infancy, it is necessary to be sure that there is not a foreign body in the eye. In the absence of a foreign body, neomycin or sulphacetamide drops would be used, and perhaps chlortetracycline or sulphacetamide ointment if the eyelids stick together at night. Sulphacetamide or penicillin ointment may sensitize the conjunctiva and may therefore appear to be ineffective.

Eye drops and eye ointment should be discarded after two weeks, because they may become infected.

The preparations used are sulphacetamide (Albucid) drops 10 per cent or 30 per cent; ointment 2½ per cent, 6 per cent or 10 per cent.

CONSTIPATION

The treatment of constipation largely depends on the cause. It is normal for the fully breast-fed baby to have infrequent stools, for instance one stool every five days, and no treatment is required. In fact the fully breast-fed baby is never constipated unless he has Hirschsprung's disease, which is rare, or intestinal obstruction.

The artificially fed baby may be constipated because he is not being given enough fluid, especially in hot weather, when he may need more than the standard 2½ oz. per lb. per day (154 ml. per kg.). He may be constipated because he is not being given sufficient sugar in the feed, or not being given enough milk. This is remedied by making up the feed properly (*e.g.* giving 2 measures of the milk powder, such as full-cream Cow and Gate, National Dried milk or Ostermilk No. 2, per lb. of body weight per day, one teaspoonful of sugar per lb. per day, with 2½ oz. (71 ml.) of water per lb. per day. If he wants more, he should have as much as he wants. An occasional baby still passes hard stools in spite of being given a correct feed. I would suggest that such a baby should be given thickened feeds, including puréed prunes or other puréed fruit. Sometimes the clinic orange juice may be sufficient to work the bowels. Some think that brown sugar works the bowels better than white sugar, but I am not sure how true this is.

It is better to deal with the constipation by correcting the feeds than by giving a laxative; but sometimes a baby in spite of everything still has hard stools which cause him discomfort, and then it is wise to give milk of magnesia, as little as is needed to make the stools normal, *e.g.* half a teaspoonful once or twice a day. The quantity should be stated clearly to the mother, for I have known two mothers who thought that milk of magnesia was a feed, and gave a whole 8-oz. bottle of it to the baby.

If an older baby (*e.g.* after 6 months) is constipated, it is usually possible to correct it by increasing the amount of fruit given, especially pears and prunes. As in the case of the younger baby, one should not allow him to continue to pass hard stools which hurt him.

From this age onwards an important cause of constipation is the deliberate withholding of stools due to overenthusiastic toilet training, the mother having compelled him to sit on the pottie against his will, or having smacked him for not using it. The baby has thus become conditioned to associate the pottie with discomfort and will not use it. He may also withhold stools because he has an anal fissure, or finds it painful to pass hard stools. It is not certain whether the fissure is the cause or the result of the constipation. It follows that the constipation must be treated by attention to the cause. An anal fissure should be treated by attending to the constipation and applying a minimal amount of an ointment which is not likely to sensitize the skin, *e.g.* plain vaseline or lignocaine ointment until it is healed.

Other substances which may be used when simple measures have failed include Senokot, bisacodyl (Dulcolax), syrup of figs, rhubarb mixture, and milk of magnesia. There are preparations of oxyphenisatin, the active principle in prunes. A recent addition is Danthron. I know of no evidence that any one of these preparations is better than any other.

When a toddler or young child presents with the story of soiling the pants and diarrhoea, by far the commonest cause is constipation. Liquid material escapes round a huge faecal mass in the rectum and leaks out of the anus. I have seen one such child treated for a prolonged period by constipating medicine – when he was already suffering from severe constipation. When on rectal examination one feels a huge faecal mass, either a bisacodyl suppository (Dulcolax) or an enema of normal saline must be given in the first place to empty the bowel. The use of water alone might be dangerous and cause water intoxication. This is then followed by liquid paraffin 3 ml./kg., increasing the dose if necessary until there are three or four stools per day. It is discontinued as soon as possible. Orange juice may be given after the paraffin to remove the unpleasant taste. The child is encouraged to eat dates, figs and prunes. He is then taught to go to the lavatory every morning after breakfast. It is useful if his feet can be on the ground when he is trying to defaecate. It is essential to see such a child at regular intervals, for relapse is common. Soiling should stop immediately the constipation has been relieved. It would be a mistake to think that the treatment is easy. In a controlled study, a stool-softening agent, dioctyl sulphosuccinate (Manoxol) was ineffective.

As for constipation in the older child, it is now well recognized that purgatives should be avoided unless they are absolutely essential. It does a child no harm to have a bowel action every other day.

Preparations

Bisacodyl (Dulcolax)
5 mg. tablets 1–5 years 1 tablet
              6–12 years 1–2 tablets at night
Suppository up to 1 year 5 mg.
            1–12 years 10 mg.
Milk of magnesia
2–4 ml. b.d.
Oxyphenisatin (Bydolax, Cirotyl, Contax)
5–10 years 1 capsule (5 mg.) at night.
Rhubarb mixture BNF paediatric
up to 1 year 5 ml.
1–5 years   10 ml.
Senna Standarized
Age 1 1·5 g. at night
Age 7 3 g.   1 level teaspoonful
Puberty 6 g. = 3 g. granules
             = 2 tablets of Senokot
Syrup of figs compound BPC
dose 2·5–10 ml.

References

ANON. (1967) Newer laxatives. *Drug and Therapeutics Bulletin*, 5, 69.
DAVIDSON M., KUGLER M.M. & BAUER C.H. (1963) Diagnosis and management in children with severe protracted constipation and obstipation. *J. Pediat.* 62, 261.
RENDLE-SHORT J. (1956) Dioctyl sodium sulphosuccinate in the treatment of constipation. *Lancet*, 2, 1189.

CONVULSIONS

Convulsions are so common in children (occurring in about 6–7 per cent of all children), and it is so essential to make the correct diagnosis in order that the correct treatment may be given, that I have decided to depart from my practice in other parts of this book and give here the main causes of convulsions and the principal differentiating features. I have discussed them in detail elsewhere (Illingworth 1971).

(1) Newborn

The common causes are hypoglycaemia, hypocalcaemia, cerebral oedema or haemorrhage, and meningitis. In some countries abroad, tetanus is a common cause. One must not guess at the diagnosis. The correct treatment is urgent in the case of hypoglycaemia, for serious brain damage may occur, and it is extremely urgent in the case of meningitis. The child should be referred to hospital immediately.

(2) Breath-holding attacks

These occur in infants and children under 5 when they are hurt or thwarted. They are rare before the age of 6 months. They are of two types – cyanotic and pallid. In the more common cyanotic type, the child cries, holds his breath in expiration, rapidly goes blue, and if he holds it for 10–15 seconds longer, he goes limp; if he holds it for still another 10 or 15 seconds, he has a major fit indistinguishable from epilepsy. The pallid type usually follows a minor injury; the child immediately becomes pale and limp. It closely resembles a faint or vasovagal attack.

It is not always easy to distinguish the breath-holding attack from epilepsy. In the breath-holding attack there is always a precipitating factor, and almost always a cry first, whereas neither is a feature of epilepsy. In a breath-holding attack cyanosis occurs at the beginning, whereas in an epileptic fit cyanosis follows the convulsion.

For treatment, see p. 104.

(3) Febrile convulsions

This is the commonest cause of fits between 6 months and 5 years, but is extremely rare after 5. It does not occur after 6. For this diagnosis, there must be a history that the child was off colour for a few hours before the fit; the fit must never last more than 10 minutes; it only occurs with the rapid rise of temperature, and never at any other time; there must not be a second fit with the same infection; the fit should not be focal. The fits are confined to the age period of about 6 months to 5 years. One difficulty in the diagnosis is the fact that fever precipitates fits in epileptics; and any severe prolonged fit itself causes a rise in temperature.

It is a mistake to make a confident diagnosis of a febrile convulsion in the home, in case the cause of the fit is pyogenic meningitis. The child should be referred to hospital.

The treatment of the actual fit is the same as that of status epilepticus (p. 160). The safest immediate treatment for the family doctor to give is paraldehyde intramuscularly (into the thigh); the child is then immediately sent to hospital.

On recovery from the convulsion, continuous antiepileptic treatment is not indicated. The parents should be told that up to the age of 5, whenever and as soon as it is decided that the child is developing another infection with a rise of temperature, he should be tepid sponged, given an aspirin, and a full dose of phenytoin and phenobarbitone (*i.e.* a dose suitable for his age) for one day only – for febrile convulsions only occur with the rapid rise of temperature.

(4) Epilepsy

Epileptic fits may occur at any age, but there are so many causes of fits in children, and the correct treatment is so dependent on a correct diagnosis, that every child with a convulsion should be referred to hospital. Apart from epilepsy one has to bear in mind the possibility of various metabolic causes, like hypoglycaemia.

A common type of fit in the infant, especially from 4 months to about 18 months, is the infantile spasm. The child may have several attacks a day; when sitting he suddenly falls forward; it is an instantaneous movement occupying a fraction of a second; it is grand mal and *not* petit mal. It is nearly always associated with mental subnormality, and treatment is frequently unsatisfactory. Early treatment may perhaps halt the process, and for that reason prompt referral to a paediatrician is advised.

Petit mal is rare before two, which immediately distinguishes it from infantile spasms; it is hardly ever associated with a change of posture or a fall – which again distinguishes it from infantile spasms; it never lasts over 20 seconds; there is a momentary staring, flicking of the eyelids, but no stiffness; there is always a characteristic EEG. It is frequently difficult to distinguish petit mal from grand mal clinically, but an EEG will establish the diagnosis. As the treatment of the two conditions is completely different, the correct diagnosis is essential.

The numerous types of grand mal will not be discussed here.

For treatment, see p. 160.

(5) Teething

Convulsions are never due to teething.

Reference

ILLINGWORTH R.S. (1971) *Common Symptoms of Disease in Children.* 3rd edn. Blackwell, Oxford.

COUGH

The treatment of cough depends on the cause. The commonest cause of a cough is a cold, and no treatment is required. Young children frequently have a troublesome cough following a cold only when they lie down in bed at night. This is due to a postnasal discharge. No medicine will affect this, but the cough may be less troublesome if the child can be induced to sleep in the prone position. In either case there is no indication for either antibiotics or a cough medicine.

Cough suppressants for the common cough following a cold, whether it is due to pharyngitis, tracheitis, bronchitis or a postnasal discharge, are contraindicated, because suppression of a cough, when there is exudate, may cause collapse of a lung. Neither is there any indication for an expectorant; the value of any expectorant is in doubt, and though theoretically potassium iodide might help it must be remembered that prolonged administration of iodides may lead to goitre formation. Bromhexine (Bisolvon) may perhaps help to liquefy thick secretions (*Drug and Therapeutics Bulletin* 1969).

There is no place for antihistamine preparations either prescribed alone or in proprietary preparations. They tend to dry secretions, and they may do more harm than good. Their only virtue is their soporific effect. In the Children's Hospital at Sheffield we do not prescribe expectorants or other cough medicines. I agree with Professor Wade (1961) who wrote about cough mixtures and linctuses in the following words: 'The use of these is hallowed by tradition. It is well to appreciate that their action is mainly that of placebos.'

It is possible that on rare occasions a 'tickling' dry cough which is troubling a child may be helped by codein linctus BPC. There is no satisfactory evidence that pholcodine or dextromethorphan BNF (Romilar) are any more effective.

If the cough is due to whooping cough, it is possible that bromhexine might help, but I have no experience of its use. No treatment is required for the cough following influenza. If the cough is due to a postnasal discharge from adenoids or from an infected antrum, these should be treated. The treatment of bronchiolitis, pneumonia and asthma is discussed in the appropriate section. There is no indication for the treatment of the cough as distinct from the cause. A cough may be due to smoking. In that case the smoking should be discouraged. A cough may be a mere tic or attention-seeking device, and no medicine is required.

A cough may be due to a foreign body in the bronchus. If there is a history of the sudden onset of a cough in a previously well child, the possibility of a foreign body must be considered, especially if it is known that the child was eating peanuts or was playing with small objects. The diagnosis certainly cannot be excluded because there is no history of the inhalation of a foreign body or of the sudden onset of a cough: in one study a history of inhalation of a foreign body was obtained in only 32 of 94 children in which this diagnosis was established. A dried pea may cause no symptoms for several hours after inhalation; the pea then swells in the bronchus and causes obstruction. The history may be deceptive, and lead to serious errors in treatment. It is a disaster to fail to make the diagnosis.

There is no doubt that there is a gross abuse of antibiotics and cough medicines for the treatment of cough. The prescription of medicine for a cough per se *in a child should be rare indeed.*

Preparation

Bromhexine (Bisolvon)
Elixir 4 mg. in 5 ml.
5–10 years Elixir 5 ml. q.d.
Under 5 years Elixir 5 ml. b.d.
8 mg. tablets; 1–2 tablets t.d.

References

ANON. (1965) Cough suppressants. *Drug and Therapeutics Bulletin*, **3**, 47.
ANON. (1969) Bisolvon. *Drug and Therapeutics Bulletin*, **7**, 89.
WADE O.L. (1961) Cough remedies. *Prescribers' Journal*, **1**, 40.

CRETINISM

It is essential that a suspected cretin should be referred immediately to hospital for establishment of the diagnosis and for treatment, with radiological and possibly biochemical control of the dosage.

The initial dose of thyroxin is low, and is rapidly built up to the optimum dose. Initial overdosage may cause heart failure and death. Overdosage at a later stage may cause tremors, nervousness and diarrhoea, but the most likely result would be excessive height increase, with advanced skeletal maturation as shown in the X-ray, followed by premature closure of the epiphyses and resulting dwarfism. Underdosage results in poor height gain and unnecessarily poor mental development.

The dose of thyroxin is 0·025 mg. b.d. increasing as indicated.

CRYING

The family doctor is likely to be asked for advice about excessive or troublesome crying in a baby. The treatment must depend on the cause, and the causes are numerous (Illingworth 1968).

The following are the most important relevant factors and causes with appropriate treatment, where possible:

(1) Personality

Some babies, however skilful the management, cry more than others. All babies are different; some are happy, smiling, placid babies, others are difficult determined characters taking after their father in that respect. All one can do, when faced with a well thriving bad-tempered baby who has nothing wrong with him, is to reassure the mother about the absence of disease or discoverable discomfort, and to explain that the baby cannot be blamed for taking after his father.

(2) Feeding problems

The cause of the crying may be hunger. Whenever discussing the feeding of a bottle-fed baby, it is essential to determine how the feed is being made up, in terms of quantity of milk powder, sugar and water. The feed being given may be too dilute, so that the baby is not receiving enough milk. The mother may fear overfeeding and so limit the food intake, much to the annoyance of her baby (and of the neighbours, who are disturbed by his crying). She may be feeding the young baby by a rigid feeding schedule, instead of letting him in the early weeks have feeds more or less when he wants them. He may be thirsty in hot weather.

The crying may be due to wind. In a breast-fed baby excessive wind is due to his sucking too long on the breast or to insufficiency of milk. No feed should take more than 10 minutes on each side; if it does, the baby is using the breast as a pacifier and is swallowing air. It is not commonly realized by mothers that all wind which troubles babies is air which they have swallowed; it is not produced in the stomach. The longer the baby takes over a feed, the more likely he is to be troubled by wind. When a baby is bottle-fed, the usual cause of excessive wind is too small a hole in the teat. Instead of taking about 10 minutes the feed takes 45–60 minutes – and all the time the baby is swallowing air. He takes too long on the feed because the hole in the teat is too small. When the bottle is inverted, the milk should almost pour out; if it does not, the hole in the teat (if the teat is a rubber one) should be enlarged by a red-hot needle (the needle having been inserted into a cork). The hole in the teat may be large enough for milk, but the mother may adopt the absurd practice of putting rusks into the bottle. Two mothers complained to me that their babies had excessive wind, and I found that they had filled the bottle with sago pudding and expected the baby to extract it through the teat. Wind may also be caused by allowing the baby to create a vacuum in the bottle by sucking the air out, so that the teat flattens and no further milk can be extracted. The air should be allowed to bubble in at frequent intervals by periodically withdrawing the teat from the baby's mouth. Similarly the baby may suffer from wind if he is allowed to suck from a bottle propped up on the pillow.

There is no need to give medicine for wind; it is a waste of money and entirely useless.

A cause of crying in older babies and young children is food forcing – trying to make the child eat when he does not want food. The mother should be told that it is never necessary to try to make a child eat.

I have had babies referred to me because of screaming at feed times. They wanted to help to hold the bottle or to feed themselves, and this was not being allowed.

Evening colic is a little understood condition. The baby has rhythmical screaming attacks in the evening, mainly between 6 p.m. and 10 p.m. (see *Colic, Evening*, p. 122). If the diagnosis is correct, it is prevented by giving a teaspoonful of the syrup of dicyclomine hydrochloride before the 6 p.m. feed.

(3) Boredom, loneliness, the desire to be picked up, jealousy

Many intelligent babies are not prepared even as young as two months of age to be left lying down with nothing to do but look at a ceiling and they cry continuously. They want to be propped up in the company of the mother in the kitchen, where they can see fascinating domestic activities. I have had many babies referred to me for crying due to simple boredom and loneliness.

Some mothers are afraid of spoiling their babies if they pick them up when they are crying. Such mothers should be assured that they will not spoil their babies by attending to their basic needs for love and comfort; they will spoil them by denying them those satisfactions. Life will be a lot easier for a mother in later months and years if she has given the baby all the love and attention which he needed in earlier days.

(4) Habit formation

The main factor in sleep problems of young children is bad habit formation (see *Sleep*, p. 241). There is no place for drugs for this, except only for a few days to help to break a well-established bad habit.

(5) The ego and negativism

Much crying is due to efforts to force the child to do things against his will – to eat, to use the pottie, to stop sucking his thumb. Crying is commonly an attention-seeking device – and often a device to get a sibling into trouble. If the mother displays great anxiety and fusses whenever the child falls, it must be expected that the child will cry excessively at the slightest graze or bump.

(6) Discomfort

The well child may be tired, cold, too hot, teething, have an itch or have a wet nappie. It is normal for well babies at about 5 or 6 months of age to cry when passing urine. They may certainly cry on passing urine if they have a nappie rash. A child may cry if he passes a hard stool.

Young babies may cry when the light is put out; others cry when the light is put on. One cannot please everyone.

The child may cry because he has a pain – in the head, in the abdomen, or in a fractured limb. When a child is poorly, crying may be due to otitis media or other infection. Other obvious causes of crying in an ill child include intussusception, appendicitis or strangulated hernia.

Metabolic conditions associated with excessive crying include phenylketonuria and coeliac disease.

A crying baby is a challenge to a family doctor, especially if the baby is ill. I would suggest that the first place to look at is the ear drum. If the child is ill and no cause can be found, he should be referred to a paediatrician forthwith; the baby may have pyogenic meningitis, a condition which in babies is commonly not associated with neck stiffness. The most dangerous diagnosis to make when an ill child is crying excessively is teething; the cause of crying is not teething if the child is ill.

If a mother wishes to give her baby a dummy or pacifier, I do not discourage it. Although the dummy is used predominantly by the lower social classes, and its use is unnecessary, and although the dummy is aesthetically offensive to many, it must be admitted that no one has shown that it does any harm – except only when the dummy is attached to a container holding sweet liquids, or is dipped into honey or other sweet substance, in which case it will have a disastrous effect on the child's teeth.

Reference

ILLINGWORTH R.S. (1968) *The Normal Child*. London, Churchill.

CYANOSIS, PERIPHERAL

Cyanosis of the arms and legs in the newborn period is normal and does not require treatment. The colour of the face, tongue and trunk is normal, so that congenital heart disease is readily eliminated.

CYANOTIC ATTACKS (Apnoeic attacks)

These have been discussed fully elsewhere (Illingworth 1971). Briefly, they are due to three groups of causes:
(1) Obstruction of the airway – by mucus, milk, regurgitated stomach contents etc.
(2) Immaturity or depression of the respiratory centre – as in oedema of the brain, prematurity, meningitis.
(3) Convulsions – of which the main causes are cerebral oedema or haemorrhage, hypoglycaemia, hypocalcaemia, severe infections.

It follows that the treatment depends on the cause. Many so-called cyanotic attacks are in reality convulsions, and as a major cause of these is hypoglycaemia, for which urgent specialized treatment is necessary, it follows that all infants with cyanotic attacks should be sent to hospital immediately. If it is obvious that the attack is merely due to milk which has entered the trachea, every effort should be made immediately to aspirate the offending material by a mucus catheter. If the child is seen when apnoeic, firm pinching of a toe or compression of the chest or artificial respiration should cause the child to make the necessary inspiration.

Reference

ILLINGWORTH R.S. (1971) *Common Symptoms of Disease in Children.* 3rd edn. Oxford, Blackwell Scientific Publications.

CYCLICAL VOMITING

See *Migraine*.

DACRYOCYSTITIS

Dacryocystitis is often associated with an incompletely open naso-lachrymal duct, with resultant stasis in the upper blind sac and predisposition to infection. As the duct nearly always opens spontaneously in a few weeks, certainly by six months, one is reluctant to have the duct probed, because this involves a general anaesthetic. It is better to try to control the infection by repeatedly massaging the duct upwards towards the eye, to drain it, together with antibiotic ointment or drops (*e.g.* neomycin).

THE DEAF CHILD

A child learns to speak by imitating the speech of others. The average age at which a child begins to say two or three words with meaning is 12 months. In the weeks preceding that he has listened to his parents and others, and has learnt the meaning of several words; all children learn the meaning of words long before they can articulate them. It is important that the deaf child should be able to hear sounds with the help of a hearing aid during these early months, and hence early diagnosis is desirable. A hearing aid can be fitted by 6 months of age, so that deafness should be diagnosed if possible by that age. Whenever a parent suspects that a child is deaf, the suspicion should be taken seriously and the child should be referred to an expert for advice. The family doctor may himself suspect deafness, on the basis of simple tests (*e.g.* crumpling paper about 18 in. from the ear, on a level with the ear, to test a child of 4 months or older, to see if he turns his head to sound).

When the specialist has diagnosed deafness, advice will be given to the parents concerning the child's management. The family doctor can help the parents to carry out the advice given.

Experts have listed the following advice to parents of a deaf child:
Talk, talk, talk to him.
Let him see you talk; see that there is light on your face.
Do not talk to him more than about four feet away; talk on a level with his face.

When you talk to him, do not move your head or your hands, because it may distract him from watching your face.

Do not exaggerate mouthing of words and lip movements.

Speak a little more slowly than usual.

Speak in a normal voice; do not shout.

Always use the words in complete sentences.

Let him feel your face as you speak – to feel the vibrations.

Act as you speak; let him see you take the shoes off, as you use the words; let him see you take a drink, wash your face, wipe your mouth, as you tell him what you are doing.

Explain constantly the happenings around the home. Talk about immediate things, so that he learns associations.

Read to him; show him pictures.

Play with him, constantly talking to him.

Help him to learn size, shape, colour, thickness, texture, depth.

Never leave him out of conversation; make him feel that he is part of the family. Invite friends to the house for him.

Teach independence, try to get him to do things for himself, to take responsibility, to help in the house. Do not do everything for him.

Repeat all the words which he has learned in the day.

Encourage interests.

Be specially sure that he feels loved, wanted, secure, important.

Be tolerant of temper tantrums when he feels thwarted in making his wants known; but exert normal loving discipline, as with any normal child.

Do not expect too much of him, especially in concentration.

Parents may be given valuable help from: The Royal National Institute for the Deaf, 105 Gower Street, London WC1.

Prevention of deafness

The family doctor plays an important part in the prevention of deafness when he makes a prompt diagnosis of otitis media and applies the appropriate treatment. Residual fluid may persist in the middle ear, however (serous otitis or glue ear), and if the hearing does not return to normal, the help of the otolaryngologist should be sought.

Recent work on the effect of loud noise in causing deafness is also of importance. The relationship between loud noise in industry and deafness is well established. It is now known that the loud noise of some modern dance halls may lead to deafness, and young people should be warned of the danger. The family doctor may contribute to the prevention of deafness by guiding young people in his practice when the opportunity presents itself.

References

BAKWIN R.M. (1950) The deaf child. *J. Pediat.* 36, 668.

DEY F.L. (1970) Auditory fatigue and predicted permanent hearing defects from rock and roll music. *New Engl. J. Med.* 282, 467.

SIR ALEX & LADY EWING (1964) *Teaching Deaf Children to Talk.* Manchester University Press.

FREEDMAN A.R. (1969) Rock'n Roll music harmful. *Clinical Pediatrics*, 8, 58.

LIPSCOMB D.M. (1969) High intensity sounds in the recreational environment. Hazards to young ears. *Clinical Pediatrics*, 8, 63.

MYKLEBUST H.R. (1950) *Your Deaf Child: A Guide for Parents.* Springfield, Charles Thomas.

RUPP R.R. & KOCH L.J. (1969) Effects of too loud music on human ears. *Clinical Pediatrics*, 8, 58.

WHETNALL E. (1956) Discussion on the management of deafness in the young child. *Proc. Roy. Soc. Med.* 49, 455.

WHETNALL E. & FRY D.B. (1964) *The Deaf Child.* London, Heinemann.

DEATH AND DYING

The management of the child with a fatal disease, the counselling of the parents as to the impact on the family, is one of the most difficult tasks that fall to a doctor. It is impossible to generalize about the matter, and one can only be guided by the age and personality of the child, the personality of the parents, the nature of the disease and numerous other factors. Evans (1969) wrote: 'I have no strategy, and tactics are improvised as events demand.' The matter is so difficult that I have appended several references to papers which seemed to me to be helpful. I am grateful to the authors of these papers for many of the comments and suggestions below.

Although the consultant usually has the task of breaking the bad news of a lethal disease when talking to the parents, the family doctor may well have the more difficult task of continued counselling and of dealing with the innumerable problems in the home; for unless, for social or other reasons, home care is out of the question, it is usually better for the child with a fatal disease to leave the hospital as soon as possible and return home. It is a matter for individual parents to decide whether they would rather that the child died in the hospital or at home. There may also be circumstances which make it necessary for the family doctor rather than the consultant to break the news to the parents.

When the news of a fatal disease is to be broken, it is better, if possible, to tell both parents together, so that one parent does not have to tell the other. This is not often possible in hospital practice, but it is likely to be easier for the family doctor to be able to talk to both together. The doctor has to decide in each case how much can be said to the parents; sometimes it is better to give all the necessary information at once, whereas in other cases it is better to break the news by degrees – in the first interview saying that the disease is serious, and giving a more accurate prognosis on the second occasion. Whatever is said, it is most unwise to put a time limit on the child's life; it never helps, and can be grossly inaccurate.

Parents may have guilt feelings, and attempt to blame themselves or someone else for the tragedy. This attitude must be anticipated, so that it may be made clear at once that neither parent is to blame. It is important not to hint at or imply blame on anyone's part, and not to suggest that earlier or different treatment could have saved the child. It is far better for the parents to feel that the tragedy was entirely unavoidable. The cause may well be unknown; if it is, they should be told so. It is most important to make it clear that everything that should have been done has been done, and that everything possible is now being done. If the parents want to know whether another child may be affected, the question must be answered; but it is better for the specialist to deal with such a question if there are possible genetic factors. Bergman & Schulte (1967) in a useful article, emphasized the importance of the physician inspiring confidence that he knows just what he is doing, of his being thorough and conscientious, of his always being available to visit when the parents are worried, of his providing continuous care, and giving personal help and attention to the child's needs with his special problems and symptoms.

The parents must be told the facts as far as they are known. They must not be allowed to expect miracles. They should certainly be encouraged to obtain a second opinion if they wish, but they should thereafter be strongly discouraged from 'shopping around' for further opinions. They must not be given any unwarranted reassurance or untrue grounds for optimism. Above all, they should be treated unhurriedly with sympathy and given ample opportunity to ask questions.

It is extremely difficult to advise the parents about what to say to the siblings. The siblings will have to be prepared for the child's death. The family doctor may have to be the one to tell them; the problem must be discussed with the parents.

The parents will need advice about the management of the child. Discipline must not be relaxed in a chronic illness, such as leukaemia, until the terminal stages, for that would cause troublesome behaviour problems. Every effort must be made to avoid favouritism to the child, for the well siblings would then suffer. Boredom must as far as possible be prevented by keeping the child occupied. If his appetite is poor, there must be no food forcing, for that will make him worse; he may be tempted by dishes which he likes: no medicine will help him.

It is important that the parents should not let the child see how anxious and disturbed they are. It is extremely difficult to avoid this, but the family doctor may help by warning them of the danger.

If the child asks whether he is going to die, one may say that one cannot say and that some recover. One does not otherwise tell a child that he is going to die. He may have fantasies about death and punishment (particularly, it is said, between the ages of 3 and 7) and these must be dealt with if possible. If he wants to talk and ask questions, he must be given the chance to ask all that he wants. It is better not to volunteer information and not to say more than he wants to know. If one conceals the outlook from the child, it is wise to conceal it from his friends also, because otherwise they are likely to convey anxiety to him by their attitudes. The child must never be put into the position of having to pretend that he does not know that he is going to die. If he is old enough to understand, he is told in advance about the necessary diagnostic and therapeutic procedures. The child and his parents may be helped and supported by their religion, and by the padre whom they know and trust.

The family doctor should certainly treat the child's symptoms, but should resist the temptation of prescribing useless medicines, particularly if they are unpleasant to take or have undesirable side effects. It would be most unfair to give injections which are useless. Pain may be relieved by pethidine or morphia. More powerful sedation may be secured by a combination of pethidine, promethazine and chlorpromazine (Evans 1968). Bone pain may be relieved by butazolidine or irradiation. Anxiety may be relieved by sodium amytal, meprobamate or prochlorperazine. As Yudkin pointed out (1967), anxiety may be manifested by depression, loss of interest in daily activities, or unprovoked anger and resentment. Sleep may be secured by pentobarbitone (Nembutal) or quinalbarbitone (Seconal).

The time may come when the child is dying, and unpleasant treatment or treatment having unpleasant side effects (*e.g.* mouth ulcers in the case of leukaemia) should be withheld. The doctor should make this decision after explaining the situation to the parents. It is unfair to expect the parents to make the decision to let the child die in peace.

When the child is finally dying, the doctor should avoid 'mock heroics' of cardiac massage and injections.

When he has died, the siblings will be told truthfully what has happened. They will already have been told that death was imminent. Children under 6 should not normally be expected to attend the funeral; over the age of 9 it may be desirable, but it is a matter of individual judgement in each case. They should not be given drugs, such as antidepressants.

The parents should be seen and supported after the child's death. Once more they may need convincing that nothing could have saved the child's life; that earlier diagnosis would not have affected the outcome; and that they did everything that they should have done for him.

The problem of helping children who have lost one of their parents is just as difficult, or more so. The effect depends partly on their age and on the duration of the parent's illness. Arthur & Kemme (1964) studied 83 disturbed children who had experienced the death of a parent; they suffered a feeling of abandonment, insecurity, worthlessness and guilt. The family doctor may have the difficult task of trying to support them after their loss.

References

ARTHUR B. & KEMME M.L. (1964) Bereavement in Childhood. *J. Child Psychol. Psychiat.* 5, 37.

BERGMAN A.B. & SCHULTE C.J.A. (1967) Care of the Child with Cancer. *Pediatrics*, 40, 487 (Symposium).

COBB, B. (1956) Psychological impact of long illness and death of a child on the family circle. *J. Pediat.* 49, 746.

EVANS A.E. (1968) If a child must die. *New Engl. J. Med.* 278, 138.

EVANS P.R. (1969) The management of fatal illness in childhood. *Proc. Roy. Soc. Med.* 62, 549.

FRIEDMAN S.B., CHODOFF P., MASON J.W. & HAMBURG D.A. (1963) Behavioral observations on parents anticipating the death of a child. *Pediatrics*, 32, 610.

SOLNIT A.J. & GREEN M. (1959) Psychologic considerations in the management of deaths in Pediatric Hospital Services. *Pediatrics*, 24, 106.

SOLNIT A.J. (1965) The dying child. *Develop. Med. Child Neurol.* 7, 693.

TOCH R. (1964) Management of the child with a fatal disease. *Clin. Pediatrics*, 3, 418.

YUDKIN S. (1967) Children and death. *Lancet*, 1, 37.

DERMAL SINUS, CONGENITAL

The routine examination of any baby includes inspection of the midline of the back for a congenital dermal sinus. If the sinus is not immediately visible, its presence may be revealed by a tuft of hair or a patch of pigmentation. Except in the upper end of the natal cleft, and unless the sinus is a blind one, a congenital dermal sinus demands surgical treatment, for if it extends into the subarachnoid space, it is extremely likely to cause pyogenic meningitis. A sinus in the upper end of the natal cleft cannot extend into the subarachnoid space, and only requires treatment if it is thought that the sinus is so long – the blind end not being visible – that infection in it is liable to occur. It may then be closed surgically at the age of 3 or 4 years.

DIABETES MELLITUS

A diabetic mother must be delivered in hospital because expert management with laboratory help is essential for the management of the baby. For instance, the baby is liable to severe hypoglycaemia, for which urgent specialist treatment is necessary. He is apt to be immature, in spite of his birthweight, and to suffer from the respiratory distress syndrome. It must be remembered that such a child is at considerable risk of developing diabetes himself in later years.

The management of a diabetic child must be under the constant supervision of a specialist. The child has to be admitted to hospital for initial stabilization, and is likely to be readmitted subsequently for restabilization if the control of the amount of glucose in the urine becomes unsatisfactory or if ketosis develops. If there is to be a change from soluble to lente insulin, readmission is desirable. If a general anaesthetic is required for dental treatment, it is safer to administer this in hospital than in the dentist's surgery. One should expect that as puberty approaches, the need for more insulin will arise.

The child should be given BCG to prevent tuberculosis, to which there is an increased susceptibility.

The commonly accepted view concerning diet is that the child should have a 'free diet without licence' – to use the words of W.W. Payne of the Children's Hospital, Great Ormond Street, London. Children vary in the amount of exercise which they take, and strict dietary control is undesirable for psychological reasons. A sugar-free urine cannot be maintained without a serious risk of hypoglycaemia, which is dangerous to life and may cause brain damage. The child should have a normal well-balanced diet with a glass of milk or a sandwich before going to bed; sweets are allowed, but (as for a normal child) they should not be unlimited; and there must be no carbohydrate excess. Shirkey wrote: 'Diabetic children require diets qualitatively and quantitatively similar to those of non-diabetic children. Control of the diabetic state by restriction of food cannot be attempted without jeopardizing growth and health. There is no longer any reason to believe that the course of diabetes is favourably influenced by special types of diet as have been prescribed in the past.'

There are still some physicians who advocate strict dietary control, with the weighing of foods. The aim of such rigidity was to prevent the development of arteriosclerosis which is usual within 10–20 years of the onset of the diabetes; but research in this country, Scandinavia and the United States has proved that rigid dieting has no beneficial effect in this regard. Experimental work with a corn oil diet with the same object was equally unsuccessful, and the diet was unpleasant and not without risks (Chance *et al.* 1969).

Insulin can be self-administered by children of 6–9 or so, depending on their intelligence and reliability, and they can also test their own urine for sugar. The site of injection, using a disposable needle if possible, has to be varied according to a definite plan in order to prevent lipoatrophy. A definite plan is used with a chart – for instance injecting the right arm, then the left arm, the left thigh and right thigh, the abdomen and buttocks, using each limb for several weeks without using the same site – placing each injection half-an-inch below the other in a vertical line, then in a new line half-an-inch away, avoiding any site of induration for several weeks. Gentle massage of an injected site after the injection helps to prevent these nodules. The child must be kept clean by daily baths, and should be taught good hygiene, including care of the finger nails.

The amount of insulin taken is increased when there is an infection, and decreased when there is vigorous exercise. When there is an infection, the increase is regulated by the amount of glycosuria, and carbohydrate is added. Insulin must *never* be stopped because a child with an infection is vomiting. Ketosis must not be allowed. The urine is tested for sugar four times a day at first, and later twice a day, discarding the overnight urine. The urine is tested for sugar by Clinitest and for acetone by Acetest or Denco test powder tablets. It is dangerous to keep the urine sugar-free; this means that he is having too much insulin and there is danger of hypoglycaemia. On the other hand continuous glycosuria (2 per cent or more) is undesirable, and calls for an increase in the amount of insulin. Wide variations in the amount of sugar, with frequent sugar-free specimens, indicate poor control.

The child and his parents will be told by the expert about the symptoms and management of hypoglycaemia. The symptoms include hunger, lassitude, vertigo, weakness, restlessness, pallor, abdominal pain, sweating, dilated pupils, fast pulse, temper tantrums and later tremor, diplopia, vomiting, headache, coma and convulsions. The child is instructed always to carry sugar tablets. If in doubt, the family doctor should give sugar or adrenaline in case of emergency.

The parents must also know about the symptoms of diabetic acidosis, for they demand immediate admission to hospital. They include nausea and vomiting, drowsiness, dry skin, a flushed face, a smell of acetone in the breath, heavy deep breathing, abdominal and sometimes generalized pains.

If there is an allergic reaction with itching, redness and erythema at the site of injection, the consultant should be asked about the use of insulin from a different species.

The family doctor has a big responsibility in treating a diabetic child. He has an important part to play in helping the child to live a normal life with a minimum of psychological disturbance. He may guide the parents about camping – telling them that the child should be allowed to go to camp if he wants, and by no means necessarily to a camp for diabetic children. The family doctor has the task, often a difficult one, of regular supervision, and of deciding at what stage expert help is required.

Parents should be encouraged to seek advice from The British Diabetic Association, 3/6 Alfred Place, London WC1.

The insulin preparations used are set out below.

	Maximum action Hours	Total duration Hours
Neutral insulin injection BP ⎫ Insulin injection BP (Soluble) ⎬	4–8	6–12
Globin zinc insulin injection BP	8–16	12–24
Insulin zinc suspension Semilente	8–12	12–16

	Maximum action Hours	Total duration Hours
Insulin zinc suspension BP Lente	4–24	24–30
Biphasic insulin injection BP (Rapitard)	4–24	18–24
Protamine zinc suspension injection BP (PZ)	10–24	24–30
Insulin zinc suspension (Ultralente)	10–24	24–30

References

Chance G.W., Albutt E.C. & Edkins S.M. (1969) Control of hyperlipidaemia in juvenile diabetes. Standard and corn oil diets compared over a period of 10 years. *Brit. Med. J.* 3, 616.

Malins, J.M. (1970) Insulins and diabetes. *Prescribers' J.* 10, 25.

Shirkey H. C. (1968) *Pediatric Therapy*. St. Louis, Mosby.

DIARRHOEA

Diarrhoea in infants and small children presents two major problems to the family doctor – the frequency of the condition, and the difficulty of deciding whether the child should be sent to hospital. Infantile gastro-enteritis is an alarming condition in the home, particularly when the doctor is pressed for time, because the child's condition may rapidly deteriorate. *Treatment or advice over the telephone is out of the question.* If a baby with diarrhoea and vomiting is seen in the morning, and it is decided that home treatment is possible, he should preferably be seen later that day, and certainly not later than the following morning. If the baby is dehydrated, with sunken eyes and loss of tissue turgor, or if diarrhoea and vomiting are severe and persisting, he should be sent to hospital immediately, because he may well need intravenous fluids. *An overweight baby may have quite severe acidosis and dehydration without apparent loss of tissue turgor, because fatty tissue is essentially water-free, and therefore there is no obvious change in the consistency of his skin. Better signs of dehydration are a dry mouth, sunken eyes and a sunken fontanelle.*

Tachypnoea is apt to be ascribed to a respiratory infection, when in fact it is due to serious acidosis. The family doctor must be on his guard

F

when an overweight baby develops a fever, or diarrhoea or vomiting; he may become seriously dehydrated without obvious signs in the skin, and when in doubt, such a child should be sent to hospital forthwith. Full-strength feeds should be replaced by half-strength milk if diarrhoea or vomiting develops in an overweight baby.

When a baby with gastroenteritis is first seen and it is decided to look after him at home, it is as well to take a rectal swab for pathogenic organisms, except when the diarrhoea is only trivial; the same applies to an older child; but it is not practical to take a swab from every case of diarrhoea in the home. The possibility of an associated infection, such as otitis media, urinary tract infection or even appendicitis, must not be forgotten. Diarrhoea is sometimes associated with intussusception.

It is the usual practice to take an affected baby off all food for 6–12 hours, giving nothing but clear fluid, and giving also the necessary electrolytes.

I am indebted to my colleague, Dr Frank Harris, for the following formula for use in the home.

Sodium chloride 1 g. per litre; Sodium lactate 2 g. per litre; Potassium chloride 1 g. per litre; Glucose 36 g. per litre.

180 ml./kg. are given in 24 hours (3 oz./lb./day). It should not be necessary to continue for over 24 hours. If he cannot retain it or diarrhoea continues he should be sent to hospital. The water should be tepid and not ice cold, for ice-cold drinks tend to increase peristalsis. Half-cream skimmed milk is started in 24 hours, if the diarrhoea is better, and as soon as possible half-cream milk is given undiluted, before finally a normal diet is restored.

The modern view is that antibiotic treatment is not only useless, but may be harmful. If the gastroenteritis (or diarrhoea in an older child) is non-specific, antibiotics are useless. If gastroenteritis is due to a pathogenic *E. coli*, antibiotics are probably useless. Neomycin could possibly help, in a dose of 100 mg./kg./day in 3 or 4 divided doses, gentamicin or colistin 10–15 mg./kg. in 3 or 4 divided doses, but many strains are drug resistant. When either drug is used, it would be discontinued in four or five days.

If the infection is due to shigella Sonne (Sonne dysentery), antibiotics should not be given unless the child is severely ill. Most strains are resistant to sulphonamides and streptomycin, and many to ampicillin and tetracycline. One might try ampicillin 100 mg./kg./day if the child is ill, but in general Sonne dysentery is a self-limiting condition and antibiotics should be avoided. It is because Sonne dysentery is a self-limiting condition that the use of antibiotics has become so firmly entrenched. An antibiotic is given, the diarrhoea clears, and the doctor is convinced that the child has got better because of the treatment. In fact the child would have got better just as quickly without the drug.

For diarrhoea due to salmonella, other than paratyphoid A, B or C, antibiotics are contraindicated unless the child is seriously ill. It has been abundantly shown that they do not shorten the course of the disease, but that they do prolong the carrier state. Sulphonamides are of no value.

There is no point in giving preparations containing kaolin or pectin. There is no evidence that they are of value. I find it impossible to believe that a teaspoonful or so of kaolin dispersed through the liquid contents of several feet of small intestine would reduce peristalsis so much that the diarrhoea is alleviated.

It is possible that the older child may be helped by diphenoxylate (Lomotil), but it is doubtful whether it is effective. Rarely acute neurological symptoms develop an hour or two after it has been given: they are relieved by nalorphine (2·5 mg. for a 2-year-old).

Chronic diarrhoea may be due to a variety of causes. Mothers frequently complain that a child has chronic diarrhoea when inspection of the stools shows that they are normal. Diarrhoea with incontinence in a well child is usually due to constipation. Many small children aged about 1–4 have chronic looseness of the stools, and yet are perfectly well and gain weight normally. This may be due to the 'irritable colon' syndrome, described by Davidson & Wasserman (1966). Mothers say that any fruit 'goes right through him'. No treatment is necessary and dietary restrictions are unavailing. Other causes include fat and carbohydrate malabsorption, and the treatment depends on the diagnosis.

It must not be forgotten that chronic diarrhoea may be a psychological symptom, arising from bullying at school or other worries.

Prevention

The prevention of diarrhoea when travelling abroad is a matter of great importance to parents of small children. The trouble is that the more certain the sunshine and heat, the less certain will be the hygiene. There are certain good rules to be observed.

Never allow the child to drink unboiled water or milk. Water should be boiled even for brushing the teeth.

Never let him eat salads, unpeeled fruit, ice-creams, cream cakes, cream dishes, ice drinks, shellfish, prepared meats.

The role of prophylactic antibiotics is, to say the least, doubtful. There may be some value in taking prophylactic Streptotriad – a mixture of streptomycin and a sulphonamide – beginning a day before arrival at the holiday place, and continuing until one has left. It is difficult to prove that it is of value, and there is certainly no evidence that it is of advantage to combine three sulphonamides. No other preparation can be recommended.

Preparations

Diphenoxylate (Lomotil)
1–3 years: 1 tablet or one 5 ml. spoonful b.d.
3–8 years: 1 tablet or one 5 ml. spoonful t.d.
8–12 years: 1 tablet or one 5 ml. spoonful q.d.

References

CHRISTIE A.B. (1967) The treatment of bacterial food poisoning. *Prescribers' Journal*, 7 104.
CUSHING A.H. (1967) Diagnosis and treatment; antibiotic therapy of infectious diarrhoea in children. *Pediatrics*, 40, 656.
DAVIDSON M. & WASSERMAN R. (1966) The irritable colon of childhood (Chronic nonspecific diarrhoea). *J. Pediat.* 69, 1027.
ROSENTSTEIN B.J. (1967) Salmonellosis in infants and children. *J. Pediat.* 70, 1.

DWARFISM

The numerous causes of dwarfism, as distinct from 'failure to thrive' have been discussed elsewhere (Illingworth 1971), and it is obvious that in most cases the possibility of treatment directed towards increasing the child's height does not arise. The two commonest factors affecting the child's height are the size of the parents and the size at birth. A small parent may have a small child. The smaller the child is at birth, especially if he were 'small for dates', the smaller he is likely to be in later years; in neither case can treatment be considered.

Certain preventable or treatable factors cause dwarfism. They are obesity, overdosage by thyroxin for hypothyroidism, adrenocortical hyperplasia, and anabolic steroids. In all cases there is initially unusual tallness, followed by premature closure of the epiphyses, so that there is eventually dwarfism or at least undue smallness in stature. The proper treatment of obesity, hypothyroidism and adrenocortical hyperplasia, and the avoidance of anabolic steroids, will do much to prevent this.

The use of anabolic steroids, *e.g.* norethandrolone (Nilevar), methandienone (Dianabol), in an attempt to increase a child's height is to be deprecated, firstly because they may have untoward side effects, such as hepatitis or virilization with enlargement of the phallus, and partly because, even if they do lead to an initial increase in height, they lead to premature closure of the epiphyses because of the androgenic effect, with the result that the child may eventually be even smaller than he would have been if he had had no treatment at all.

The prolonged use of corticosteroids for asthma or rheumatoid arthritis is also likely to cause stunting of growth. Intermittent dosage of prednisolone (*e.g.* 3 days a week), or the use of ACTH or tetracosactrin, may help to prevent this effect on the height. Severe asthma may itself cause stunting of growth, and more efficient treatment on the lines suggested on p. 86 may help in this way.

References

ANON. (1962) The anabolic androgenic steroids. *The Medical Letter*, **1**, 38.
ILLINGWORTH R.S. (1971) *Common Symptoms of Disease in Children*. 3rd edn. Oxford. Blackwell Scientific Publications.

DYSENTERY

See *Diarrhoea*.

DYSLALIA (Indistinct speech)

When a mother becomes worried about her child's indistinct speech, the family doctor has to decide at what stage to refer the child to a specialist. He must decide whether the child's speech is normal for his age, or normal for his mental age if he is backward, or whether he should have grown out of his baby language and requires treatment. It will be realized that if the child was late in beginning to speak, he may well be late in speaking clearly. In general, it is wise to refer a child to a paediatrician if by his fourth birthday he is speaking indistinctly. Even before that, if there is a severe speech defect, it would be wise to have the hearing tested. It is a mistake to wait until the child starts school, and is then teased for his bad speech, though it is true that many types of speech defects resolve as the child matures. The speech therapist can cure a lisp and certain other speech defects (including that associated with nasal escape). A lisp may persist if untreated.

When a child is referred to the paediatrician for his speech defect, his hearing will be tested in case there is an unrecognized high-tone deafness which is responsible for it; and the speech therapist will assess the child phonetically, and investigate the tongue, lip and palate movements.

Reference

COURT D. & HARRIS M. (1965) Speech disorders in children. *Brit. Med. J.* 2, 345, 409

DYSLEXIA (Delayed reading)

The treatment of dyslexia or delayed reading depends on the cause, and the help of a psychologist is essential to establish the diagnosis. The commonest cause of delayed reading is mental backwardness. Other causes include poor teaching and emotional factors.

The so-called 'specific dyslexia', an example of 'specific learning disorders' has been the subject of many books and articles, and reference to these has been made in my book, *The Development of the Infant and Young Child: Normal and Abnormal* (Illingworth 1970). There is almost invariably a family history of the same complaint, usually with ambidexterity, left-handedness, clumsiness, persistent reversal of symbols, and delayed speech. Treatment usually consists of combining the visual, auditory, sensory and kinaesthetic senses – so that the child sees the letters or words, hears the word pronounced and feels the words (plastic) as he speaks them. It is difficult to find an expert who gives this treatment. It is uncertain how much of any improvement which occurs is due to the treatment and how much is due to the child's maturation with age.

References

CRITCHLEY M. (1964) *Developmental Dyslexia*. London, Heinemann.

FLOWER R.M., HOFMAN H.F. & LAWSON L.I. (1965) *Reading Disorders*. Philadelphia, Davis.

FRANKLIN A.W. (1962) *Word Blindness or Specific Developmental Dyslexia*. London, Pitman.

HERMANN K. (1959) *Reading Disability* (Dyslexia). Copenhagen, Munksgaard.

ILLINGWORTH R.S. (1970) *The Development of the Infant and Young Child: Normal and Abnormal*. 4th edn. London, Livingstone.

INGRAM T.T.S. (1963) Delayed development of speech with special reference to dyslexia. *Proc. Roy. Soc. Med.* **56**, 199.

MONEY J. (1962) *Reading Disability*. Baltimore, Johns Hopkins Press.

DYSMENORRHOEA

Dysmenorrhoea is not usual in the preovulatory phase of early adolescence. It may arise from unfortunate attitudes to menstruation implanted by the mother or friends, and the family doctor can do more than anyone to reassure the girl. This is usually enough. If the dysmenorrhoea persists and is troublesome, a specialist should be consulted.

Reference

DEWHURST C.J. (1963) *Gynaecological Disorders of Infants and Children*. London, Cassell.

DYSPHAGIA

Dysphagia in the newborn baby is a complex problem, which I have reviewed elsewhere (Illingworth 1969). A child with dysphagia should be referred to a paediatrician.

Reference

ILLINGWORTH R.S. (1969) Sucking and swallowing difficulties in infancy. Diagnostic problems of dysphagia. *Arch. Dis. Childh.* **44**, 655.

EAR, FOREIGN BODY IN

The family doctor should be cautious about attempting to remove a foreign body from the ear. The task may be easy, but it is apt to be much more difficult than he expects. There have been many instances of damage to the ear drum and internal ear from enthusiastic attempts to remove a foreign body from the ear. If the object cannot be removed readily by forceps or gentle syringing, the child should be referred to a hospital, where a general anaesthetic may be given in order that the procedure will be easier. If the foreign body is paper, syringing would be unwise, because the paper would soften and be more difficult to remove.

After a foreign body has been removed from the ear, the drum should be examined to make sure that it has not been damaged.

EARS, WAX IN

There are various wax softeners on the market, including cerumol and xerumenex. They may help, but it is uncertain whether these or other preparations are any better than a vegetable oil for the purpose. Troublesome wax can usually be removed by simple syringing without prior preparation, and special drops are unnecessary; yet vast numbers of prescriptions are written annually for wax softeners at great expense to the country.

ECZEMA, INFANTILE

General comments

Severe infantile eczema is an extremely troublesome condition for mother and child. The family doctor has to be prepared to allay the mother's anxieties, remove if possible any feeling of guilt, and if necessary give her sedatives. Mothers may transfer some of their anxiety to a child, and hence the importance of treating the mother. She must be induced to avoid over-protecting or spoiling him, and should be persuaded to treat him as far as possible as a normal child.

It is better if a baby in an allergic family is fully breast-fed for the first five or six months, as he is probably less likely to become allergic to human milk than to cow's milk. Highly allergenic foods like egg should be avoided at least for six months. It would be sensible to avoid woollen clothes for a child with eczema and to try to stop him crawling on a woollen rug. If a child has eczema, the bedroom should be treated in the same way as in the case of asthma, and allergens should be avoided.

If it is thought that the eczema is due to milk allergy, Velactin or milk substitute, or soya preparations should be used instead. I think that it is likely to help only an occasional child.

Eczema may be aggravated by soap and water. In that case the child can be cleaned with ung. emulsificans instead of soap.

Admission to hospital should be avoided if possible. A child with eczema is highly susceptible to streptococcal infections of the skin, and such infections are less likely in the home.

When a child has infantile eczema, vaccination against smallpox is absolutely contraindicated. It would be likely to result in generalized vaccinia, which may be fatal. Likewise a child with infantile eczema should not be allowed to come into contact with herpes, or with another recently vaccinated child. Immunization against other conditions is not contra-indicated.

When the family doctor is discussing the problem of eczema with the parents, he will not raise the question of the commonly associated condi-tion, asthma. In case the parents should ask about it, it is as well for him to know that 40 per cent of children with eczema will develop asthma.

Specific treatment

For the common mild eczema on the face of the young baby, 1 per cent hydrocortisone ointment is effective. It should be used as sparingly as possible, three or four times a day. There are so many corticosteroid preparations for the skin that it has been impossible for anyone to carry out proper tests of their relative effectiveness. Most statements about the superior qualities of one preparation are based purely on clinical impres-sion. In my experience 1 per cent hydrocortisone ointment has proved effective for most cases, but I cannot say that other preparations would not be better or worse. Betamethasone valerate (Betnovate) or fluocinolone acetonide (Synalar) are more potent steroid preparations suitable for resistant cases, but there is a danger from their absorption, and prolonged use may cause dermal atrophy. No steroid should be used for more than a week or two at a time.

For dry eczematous lesions elsewhere, an ointment containing 1–2 per cent crude coal tar in zinc ointment is satisfactory, as is zinc paste and ichthammol bandage BPC. Subsequently Boots E.45 emollient applied at night helps to keep the skin soft. For limbs, coal tar occlusive bandages covered with tube gauze, left in place for a week, are useful and make restraints unnecessary.

For chronic lichenified lesions, crude coal tar ½–6 per cent in Lassar's paste is effective, as is crude coal tar of the same strength in zinc oxide ointment. (Coal tar preparations tend to be unpopular with parents, because of the colour.) Crusts are removed by equal parts of emplastrum plumbi BPC and paraffinum molle on lint strips left in place for 24 hours. Corticosteroid ointment may then be applied, but in using it over any large area there is a danger of absorption.

When eczema is oozing, mild agents must be employed. It is wise to begin with a saline lotion, lotio terra silica, calamine lotion or lotio aluminium acetate (BNF), until acute symptoms have subsided; thereafter it is wise to use a paste rather than an ointment (*e.g.* zinc oxide pates).

When eczema is infected, a chlorhexidine lotion (Hibitane) or cream may be used to clear up the infection, or, provided that it is only used for a week or so, one could use a steroid ointment combined with an antibiotic, such as Betnovate A. It is wise to avoid other antibiotic creams or ointment, because they sensitize the skin. When the infection has been cleared, hydrocortisone ointment may be used.

Severe itching may be reduced by diphenhydramine (Benadryl) 7·5–15 mg. three times a day for an infant, or promethazine (Phenergan) 5–10 mg. three times a day. These are useful sedatives for the night. Alternatives are trimeprazine (Vallergan) or methdilazine (Dilosyn). There is no evidence that any one antihistamine is better for the purpose than any other. Chloral 60 mg. 4-hourly may also be used. Antihistamine ointments should never be used, because they sensitize the skin.

Hydrocortisone is the cheapest and recommended corticosteroid preparation except for the rare case in which a stronger preparation, such as betamethasone valerate (Betnovate), is required; this should not be used for more than a week because of the risk of dermal atrophy. Below is a list of some of the corticosteroid ointments, for reference purposes; but it is hoped that the preparation normally used will be the hydrocortisone cream or ointment.

Corticosteroid ointments or creams

NAME	CONSTITUENTS
Adcortyl	Triamcinolone
Betnovate	Betamethazone
Betnovate A	Betamethazone with chlortetracycline
Betnovate C	Betamethazone with clioquinol
Betnovate N	Betamethazone with neomycin
Eurax HC	Hydrocortisone with crotamiton
Fucidin H	Hydrocortisone with sodium fusidate
Hydrocortisone	BP
Hydroderm	Hydrocortisone, neomycin, bacitracin
Locorten	Flumethazone
Locorten N	Flumethazone with neomycin
Neocortef	Hydrocortisone with neomycin
Propaderm	Beclomethasone
Propaderm A	Beclomethasone with chlortetracycline
Remiderm	Triamcinolone acetonide
Synalar	Fluocinolone acetonide
Synalar N	Fluocinolone with neomycin
Vioform hydrocortisone	Hydrocortisone with iodochlorhydroxyquinolone (Clioquinol)

References

JARRETT A. (1969) Corticosteroids in skin disease. *Prescribers' Journal*, 9, 15.
PERLMAN H.H. (1960) *Pediatric Dermatology*. Chicago, Year Book Publishers.
SNEDDON I.B. & CHURCH R.E. (1964) *Practical Dermatology*. London, Arnold.

ENCOPRESIS

See *Constipation*.

ENURESIS

Few subjects promote such heated disagreement amongst paediatricians and psychiatrists as does enuresis. Psychiatrists are apt to claim that enuresis is entirely psychological in origin, while paediatricians have other views.

It seems obvious to me that there are numerous causes of enuresis, often acting in association with each other. I regard primary enuresis, in which a child has never been dry, as mainly due to delayed maturation of the relevant part of the nervous system. There is nearly always a family history of the same complaint. Just as some children are later than others in sitting, walking or talking, others are later than others in controlling the bladder. There can be no doubt that sociopsychological factors are also relevant, for enuresis is more common in the lower social classes than in the upper ones; and the age at which toilet training is commenced and the way in which it is carried out are highly relevant. No one could deny that psychological problems are commonly superimposed on the main problem, that of delayed maturation.

Secondary enuresis, developing in a child who has been dry at night for a prolonged period, is nearly always psychological in origin, resulting from some form of insecurity, especially in a child who has recently acquired control of the bladder; but it may also be due to the development of frequency or polyuria in a child who has recently acquired control. Daytime wetting, certainly at school age, is usually psychological in origin unless there is constant dribbling.

Organic enuresis consists of constant dribbling incontinence, day and night. In a boy this is usually due to urethral obstruction, while in a girl it is due to an ectopic ureter entering the vagina or urethra. A good review of the surgical causes of enuresis is that of Smith (1967).

It is obvious that the treatment of enuresis must depend on the cause.

Primary enuresis

It is essential that the mother should stop scolding the child or otherwise punishing him for wetting the bed. It is useless to instruct her to limit the child's fluid intake in the evenings; it does not help. In fact Hägglund (1965) showed that it is better to increase the fluid intake of enuretics, in order that the bladder can be expanded. Some advocate, for the same reason, that children should be taught to hold the urine longer and longer during the day.

It is useful to ask when the child wets the bed. If he is dry when lifted out in the late evening, and only wet in the morning, it may be possible to keep him dry throughout the night by awakening him by means of an alarm clock in the early hours of the morning. The more usual story is that the child wets himself almost as soon as he goes to sleep.

It is customary to culture the urine before instituting treatment, but in fact there is not much association between urinary tract infection and primary enuresis.

Of the scores of drugs which have been used for bed wetting, only three deserve discussion. They are amphetamine and the tricyclic anti-depressants imipramine and amitriptyline. Amphetamine works only by reducing the depth of sleep and keeping the child awake, and so it is not useful by itself. Imipramine is widely used. In a review of its use, it was stated that 10–20 per cent of children fail to respond, 25 per cent are cured, and that the rest improve but are apt to relapse. It was thought that there was little point in trying amitriptyline if imipramine failed. It is my practice to commence treatment with imipramine in a dose of 25 mg. at night for a week; if that is not successful I prescribe 50 mg. at night; and after the age of 7 or 8 years, if that fails I prescribe 75 mg. at night, but no more. It is important to note that there are numerous possible side effects of imipramine (p. 34), and that the effective dose is close to the toxic dose. I personally have not seen side effects from thera-peutic doses, but they are well recognized. A gross overdose may cause serious myocardial damage. Because of the numerous possible side effects, it is wise to discontinue the drug as soon as possible. I would not try amitriptyline (or nortriptyline) if imipramine failed. I would not use either drug under the age of 5.

The most effective treatment for primary enuresis is the electric buzzer, curing some 66 per cent (Forsythe & Redmond 1970). The child sleeps on a special pad, and as soon as the child wets, the circuit is broken, and the buzzer sounds. The child then has to get out of bed to turn the buzzer off – and to pass urine. It should not be used for a child below the age of 5.

The buzzer often fails for the following reasons:

(1) It does not awaken the child. In that case one prescribes amphetamine 10 mg. at night to reduce the depth of sleep, or else one obtains a louder buzzer.

(2) The child is able to turn the buzzer off without getting out of bed.

He then does not empty the bladder, goes to sleep and wets the bed again.

(3) The buzzer is not used for a long enough time. It should be used for not less than two or three months. The child should be dry at night for at least three or four weeks before it is switched off. There is then much to be said for allowing the child to sleep on the pad which has been disconnected without him knowing it.

The family doctor should know that the electric buzzer may cause trouble if not properly used (Neal & Coote 1969). The wiring should be done by an expert. Misaligned foils in a disarranged bed, due to careless checking or maltreatment of the pad, may lead to ulceration of the skin and scarring, or direct current electrolysis through the moist skin.

Electric buzzers can be obtained from the following sources:
Down Bros. and Mayer & Phelps Ltd,
Church Path,
Mitcham,
Surrey;
Wessex Medical Equipment Co,
Twyford,
Winchester,
Hants;
Astric Products Ltd,
261 Queens Park Road,
Brighton,
Sussex;
N.H. Eastwood and Son Ltd,
48A Eversley Park Road,
Winchmore Hill,
London N21.

McConaghy (1969) conducted a controlled trial of imipramine, amphetamine and the buzzer; amphetamine was of little use; the buzzer was the most effective treatment initially and on follow up. Unfortunately McConaghy used a dose of imipramine (10–25 mg.) which I regard as too small to be effective.

Secondary enuresis

In case of secondary enuresis, it is essential to examine the urine for albumin, sugar, the specific gravity and evidence of infection, in order to eliminate organic conditions causing frequency and polyuria. If these are found they must be treated. Having eliminated these, one has to try to determine any cause for psychological disturbance, such as worries at home or school, bullying, unkindness, jealousy or excessive strictness. The treatment is then treatment of the cause, and if the family doctor cannot discover and treat this, he should seek the help of a child psychiatrist or paediatrician. Sometimes the cause is untreatable – for instance, a bereavement. The treatment of daytime wetting is likely to prove difficult.

The doctor must be alive to the possibility of organic causes for wetting. It is easy to ask whether there is constant dribbling incontinence, day and night. If there is, the child must be referred to a paediatrician for full investigation and for surgical treatment if the organic cause is confirmed.

Note

The NF Imipramine is cheaper than the proprietary Tofranil. Amitriptyline appears under three trade names: Triptizole, Saroten, Laroxyl.

References

ANON. (1967) Treatment of enuresis with psychoactive drugs. *Drug and Therapeutics Bulletin*, **5**, 17.

BORRIE P. & FENTON J.C.B. (1966) Buzzer ulcers. *Brit. Med. J.* **2**, 151.

FORSYTHE W.I. & REDMOND A. (1970) Enuresis and the electric alarm. Study of 200 cases. *Brit. Med. J.* **1**, 211.

HÄGGLUND T.B. (1965) Enuretic children treated with fluid restriction or forced drinking. *Ann. Paed. Fenniae*. **11**, 84.

McCONAGHY N. (1969) A controlled trial of imipramine, amphetamine, pad and bell conditioning and random awakening in the treatment of nocturnal enuresis. *M. J. Australia*, **2**, 237.

NEAL B.W. & COOTE M.A. (1969) Hazards of enuresis alarms. *Arch. Dis. Childh.* **44**, 651.

SMITH E.D. (1967) Diagnosis and management of the child with wetting. *Australian Paediatric J.* **3**, 193.

EPIGLOTTITIS

The acute onset of stridor with fever and malaise always requires prompt referral to hospital. Acute epiglottitis is usually due to the haemophilus influenzae. Obstruction may develop with alarming suddenness, and it would be most dangerous to treat such a child at home. If, when examining the child, the red swollen epiglottis is seen, the doctor should take the child to hospital himself, leaving a member of the family to telephone to the Children's ward, giving the doctor's diagnosis of epiglottitis. The antibiotic commonly recommended is ampicillin.

See also *Laryngotracheobronchitis*.

EPILEPSY

In my experience the treatment of epilepsy is frequently incorrect or at least inadequate. There are numerous causes of fits in children, and the diagnosis is not easy. In addition, the treatment for fits due to one cause is often quite unsuitable for fits due to another cause, and the treatment for one type of fit (*e.g.* petit mal) is inappropriate and in fact useless for another type (*e.g.* grand mal). It would be disastrous to treat a child for epilepsy when his fits are due to hypoglycaemia; and one has seen numerous tragedies from ascribing fits to teething (a diagnosis which is always wrong) when in fact they are due to pyogenic meningitis. Hence, before treatment is instituted, the diagnosis should be established by an expert with the necessary laboratory help.

In this section I am assuming that the diagnosis of idiopathic epilepsy is correct, and that the convulsions are not febrile fits, breath-holding attacks, or any other definable condition.

Drug treatment

All the drugs used in the treatment of epilepsy have troublesome side effects. These are listed in the section commencing on p. 30. It would be wrong to enumerate all these to parents when instituting treatment; they would cause so much anxiety, and if the child heard about them, symptoms might develop by suggestion. It may be right to say that a child may become unsteady when treated by phenytoin, and that the gums may become swollen; but otherwise I would say nothing when instituting treatment.

When a child has ordinary grand mal epilepsy but not infantile spasms, and when his intelligence is normal and he does not suffer from cerebral palsy, I tell the mother that one ought to be able to stop the fits, but that it is usually necessary to change the dosage and drugs used and to try different combinations of drugs before the child becomes fit free, as there is no one drug which will stop fits in all children. If the child is mentally subnormal or has cerebral palsy, I tell the mother that it will be difficult to stop the fits, but that one will hope to reduce their frequency and severity.

The usual plan is to commence treatment with either phenobarbitone or phenytoin. Phenobarbitone tends to have fewer troublesome side effects, but is slightly less effective than phenytoin; but phenobarbitone alone is often sufficient to prevent further fits. There is a tendency to underdose with phenobarbitone. At 2 years of age one would begin with 30 mg. twice a day.

The aim should be to alter the treatment each time a fit occurs (unless the fits are very frequent). One increases the dose of phenobarbitone until either the fits stop or side effects occur. If the side effect is drowsiness, it may be controlled by adding amphetamine. If a rash develops, the drug should be discontinued altogether.

It is not my practice to have blood barbiturate levels estimated, because one relies on the symptoms for regulating the dosage; but it is easy to give an overdose, causing excessive drowsiness and poor concentration and performance at school. (The blood level which is satisfactory is 2–3 mg./100 ml.; at a level of 5 mg./100 ml., drowsiness is usual; a level of 7 mg./100 ml. is dangerous.) Overdosage with antiepileptic drugs is common.

If fits still occur when the maximum dose is being given, phenytoin is added, the dose of that drug being increased if necessary. If fits still occur, one might add a third drug, such as phensuximide. One cannot combine primidone and phenobarbitone, because the combination is likely to cause drowsiness, for primidone breaks down to a barbiturate. Primidone can safely be combined with phenytoin, phensuximide or other drug.

If the above drugs fail, useful remaining drugs are sulthiame, diazepam, carbamazepine or pheneturide. Potassium bromide must not be discarded as useless; in conjunction with phenytoin and phenobarbitone it may be successful in stopping fits. The serum bromide level should be estimated fairly frequently, *e.g.* once every two weeks or so, aiming at a level of 150–200 mg. per 100 ml. This level is not likely to be reached for two or three weeks, though salt restriction may help. A dose of 5–10 mg. three times a day for a child under 6, or 10–15 mg. three times a day for an older child, is the usual dose. Side effects are likely to be relieved rapidly by discontinuing the drug and adding salt.

Sulthiame or carbamazepine are the drugs of choice for temporal lobe epilepsy. Sulthiame is often especially useful in the case of children who are retarded or have cerebral palsy.

Suggested scheme, to be tried in order, increasing the dosage to the maximum in each case or to the point where side effects occur;

Phenobarbitone

Phenytoin

Phenobarbitone + phenytoin

Phenobarbitone + phenytoin + phensuximide

Primidone + phenytoin

Primidone + phensuximide

Phenytoin + phenobarbitone + bromide

Phenytoin + sulthiame

Phenytoin or phenobarbitone + carbamazepine

Pheneturide

or similar combinations, but *not* primidone + phenobarbitone.

Acetazolamide or a ketogenic diet may help when other methods fail; but the diet is unpleasant and expensive, and has to be controlled with laboratory help. Acetazolamide has now largely replaced the ketogenic diet.

For any child with grand mal epilepsy, the timing of the dose should be adjusted to the child's needs. A common time for a fit is on going to sleep or on awakening. It is difficult to deal with the latter. One tries the effect of phenobarbitone spansules 60 mg. last thing at night; this is a long-acting preparation. If that is unsuccessful it may be necessary to awaken the child in the middle of the night, *e.g.* 2–3 a.m., to give a dose of phenytoin or other drug. If fits occur predominantly in the late evening, one will adjust the dose accordingly.

It should be remembered that a common cause of the continuance of convulsive episodes, despite the prescription of suitable drugs, is failure of the parents to administer the drugs. Sometimes they leave this to a young child without supervision.

For infantile spasms the treatment is unsatisfactory, and the paediatrician should be consulted. Infantile spasms are not petit mal, and hence ethosuccimide is useless. The usual initial treatment is prednisolone, corticotrophin (ACTH) or tetracosactrin, giving the corticosteroid for not more than eight weeks. If that fails one would use nitrazepam (mogadon) or any of the drugs used for grand mal, usually in combination; but one is unlikely to stop the fits. The infantile spasms usually stop spontaneously between 15 months and 24 months, but major fits may subsequently develop.

Status epilepticus. When a family doctor is faced with a child who is still convulsing, he should arrange immediately for urgent transfer to hospital, because a prolonged fit damages the brain and is dangerous. In the meantime he can safely give intramuscular paraldehyde 1 ml. per year of age, up to a maximum of 5 ml., intramuscularly, using a glass syringe, not a plastic one. In hospital it is usual to administer diazepam 2·5–10 mg. intravenously slowly over a period of 1–10 minutes, or the same dose intramuscularly; but diazepam is probably not as safe as paraldehyde, tending more to cause respiratory depression.

In addition the doctor must see that there is an airway, sucking the child out if necessary.

Petit mal

In this section I am assuming that the diagnosis is correct, and has been confirmed by the typical EEG. The EEG must be typical before the diagnosis can be accepted. The fit must not last more than 20 seconds, and there must be no twitching. A fall or change of posture is definitely rare and makes the diagnosis unlikely. It is extremely rare in the first year, and is unlikely in mentally or physically handicapped children. It is essential to make the correct diagnosis, because phenobarbitone and phenytoin are ineffective against petit mal, while the drug of choice for petit mal, ethosuccimide, is ineffective against grand mal. One must not promise to stop the fits, but one can reduce them in frequency and in two out of three children one may almost completely stop them. If the child has only an occasional attack, one has to decide whether it is worth treating at all – balancing the effect of the fit against the risk of side effects. If the attacks are only infrequent (*e.g.* seen only once every day or two) it may be unwise to increase the dose of ethosuccimide or other drug beyond the usual level, thus increasing the risk of side effects. One has to make up one's mind as to whether a few petit mal attacks are preferable to the risk of unpleasant side effects of drugs.

The drug of choice is ethosuccimide. If that fails after increasing the dose one may add phensuximide, which is less effective. Other drugs which may be tried are diazepam, acetazolamide, chlordiazepoxide, meprobamate or mepacrine. Acetazolamide has now replaced the ketogenic diet, which was at one time recommended for intractable petit mal.

Troxidone is used if other drugs fail. It is troublesome to use because of the serious side effects. Regular fortnightly blood counts are necessary.

Duration of treatment

There is no rigid rule about this. It is usual to continue treatment for two years after the last fit, and then to reduce the dose over a month or two before stopping it, restarting if a further fit occurs, which is unusual.

The treatment of the whole child

There is more in the treatment of epilepsy than the administration of drugs. The family doctor may be asked for advice about the restriction of the child's normal activities. It is important that as far as possible he should be treated as a normal child. Certainly if the fits are under control, he should be allowed to swim, provided that there is a teacher supervising who is aware that the child has had fits; but it would be unwise for him to climb on to the highest diving board, to climb high trees, or to ride a bicycle on a busy road. He should be allowed to go to school alone, if old enough, without being escorted by his parents. The question of whether he should be allowed to ride a bicycle or a horse must depend on the degree of control of fits and their severity. In general it is better for the head teacher to be aware of the diagnosis. If the drug has to be taken three times a day, a teacher may be required to see that a child takes the tablets. For the purposes of physical training and swimming lessons, the teacher must know about the diagnosis.

The child with epilepsy is apt to have troublesome educational problems. They include side effects of drugs, such as phenobarbitone, which may cause drowsiness or defective concentration; absence or exclusion from school; the psychological effect of being known to have fits and of being treated differently from other children; and interruption of the child's attention in class, as a result of frequent fits, especially petit mal.

Livingston (1970) in the United States, has reviewed the psychological problems of the epileptic child. He wrote: 'The most serious hazard of an epileptic disorder is frequently not the seizures *per se*, but the associated emotional disturbances which are prone to develop in a youngster as a result of mismanagement by his family, by his classmates and friends and by society.' He emphasized the importance of trying to obtain complete control of the fits, and of helping him to adjust to his illness and to the attitudes of others. He drew attention to the feeling of guilt which parents are apt to feel, and the importance of explaining to them that it is no fault of theirs. He advocated that the methods of treatment, the hazards and complications of treatment, and the usual course and prognosis should be explained. They should be told that many famous people suffered from epilepsy; in our book, *Lessons from Childhood* (1966) about the childhood of famous people, we listed many of them, including Alexander the Great, Petrarch, Pythagoras, Empedocles, Democritus, Julius Caesar, Alfred the Great, William III, Peter the Great, Charles V of Spain, Louis XIII, Napoleon, Archduke Charles of Austria, Richelieu, Pascal, Swedenborg, Paganini, Swinburne, Dostoevsky, Edward Lear, William Morris and Van Gogh.

It has not been my practice to use the word 'epilepsy' when talking to the parents about the diagnosis, unless they ask whether the child has epilepsy. Others think that one should be completely honest with them about the nature of the disease. Livingston advised that in the early teens the adolescent should be told about the full implications of the condition; at that age he can best understand and accept the situation.

The family doctor may be asked for genetic advice. He would be safe in saying that the genetic risk to a patient's child, when the patient is an adult, is a very small one – not more than about 1 in 25.

The family doctor should warn the parents not to leave the drugs in charge of a young child; there is always the risk of an accidental (or deliberate) overdose.

Summary

The first essential is to make the correct diagnosis. Many fits are ascribed to petit mal, for which ethosuccimide is the drug of choice and for which phenobarbitone is of no use, whereas in fact the diagnosis is grand mal, for which the drug of choice is phenobarbitone or phenytoin.

It is important for the sake of the child and for his parents to try one's best to stop fits. It is not sufficient merely to prescribe phenobarbitone 30 mg. twice a day and to adhere to that dose, however many fits the child has. Different doses and combinations of drugs should be tried. Once the diagnosis has been established, even if the child has had only one fit, treatment should be instituted and maintained for at least two years after the last fit. An epileptic fit is terrifying for parents, and severe fits may damage the brain. Determined efforts must be made to stop them.

The important psychological and educational aspects of epilepsy must not be ignored. The doctor must know about the possible side effects, including rarely the action on the blood.

Note

Phenytoin NF the official name, is less expensive than Epanutin, the proprietary name.
Parents may receive useful advice from:
The British Epilepsy Association,
3–6 Alfred Place,
London WC1.

Preparations and doses

Acetazolamide (Diamox): 250 mg. tablets, 125–250 mg. t.d.
Age 1   125 mg. b.d.
Age 7   250 mg. b.d.
Puberty   500 mg. b.d.

Carbamazepine (Tegretol): 200 mg. tablets.
2 weeks to 1 year   10 mg./kg. t.d.
1 year upwards   100 mg. t.d.
7 years   200 mg. t.d.

Ethosuccimide (Zarontin, Emeside): 250 mg. capsules, syrup 250 mg. in 5 ml.
Age 1   125 mg. t.d.
Age 7   250 mg. t.d.
Puberty   500 mg. t.d.

Nitrazepam (Mogadon): 5 mg. tablets.
2 weeks to 1 year   0·1 to 0·7 mg./kilo./day.

Pheneturide (Benuride)
½–1 year   50 mg. b.d.
1–5 years   100–200 mg. t.d.
5–10 years   200 mg. b.d. to t.d.

Phenobarbitone (Luminal): prescribe as phenobarbitone.
Infant   15 mg. b.d.
1 year upwards 30 mg. b.d.
Spansule   60 mg. at night.

Phensuximide (Milontin): capsules 250 or 500 mg.
Up to 5 years   250 mg. per day to 250 mg. q.d.
6–12 years   500 mg. per day, increasing.

Phenytoin (Epanutin): 50 mg. or 100 mg. capsules.
Up to 5 years   30 mg. t.d. increasing to 50 mg. t.d.
Suspension (30 mg. in 5 ml.)
6–12 years   50 mg. b.d. increasing to 100 mg. t.d.

Potassium bromide
Under 6 years   5–10 mg. t.d.
Over 6 years   10–15 mg. t.d.
(watch serum bromide level)

Primidone (Mysoline): 250 mg. tablets, suspension (250 mg. in 5 ml.)
Age 1   62·5 mg. t.d.
Age 7   125 mg. t.d.
Puberty   250 mg. t.d.

Sulthiame (Ospolot): 50 mg. or 200 mg. tablets.
Age 1   50 mg. t.d.
Age 7   100 mg. t.d.
Puberty   200 mg. t.d.

References

ILLINGWORTH R.S. & ILLINGWORTH C.M. (1966) *Lessons from Childhood: Some Aspects of the Early Life of Unusual Men and Women.* London, Livingstone.
KEITH H.M. (1967) *Convulsive Disorders in Children.* Boston, Little Brown and Co.
LENNOX W.G. (1960) *Epilepsy and Related Disorders.* London, Churchill.
LIVINGSTON S. (1954) *Convulsive Disorders in Children.* Springfield, Charles Thomas.
LIVINGSTON S. (1966) *Drug Therapy for Epilepsy.* Springfield, Charles Thomas.
LIVINGSTON S. (1970) The physician's role in guiding the epileptic child and his parents. *Am. J. Dis. Child.* 119, 99.
MILLICHAP G. (1967) Petit mal. *Ped. Clinics N. America,* 14, 905.

EPIPHORA (Watering of the eyes)

Few babies shed tears in the first three or four weeks. Thereafter one or both eyes may 'water' due to failure of the nasolachrymal duct (tear duct) to open. In almost all cases this will open if left alone – nearly always by the age of five or six months. Probing the duct involves the use of a general anaesthetic, and every general anaesthetic involves a small risk; probing, therefore, should not be resorted to unless it is absolutely necessary.

Sometimes an infection occurs as a result of stasis in the upper blind sac (see *Dacryocystitis*). This can usually be controlled by antibiotic eye drops (*e.g.* chloramphenicol) and repeated massage of the duct upwards towards the eye. It may be wise to massage the duct upwards towards the eye in this way not only for the treatment of infection, but also in an attempt to prevent it.

I would not use drops other than antibiotics – and they are used only when there is an infection.

EPISTAXIS

Nose-bleeding originates in well over 90 per cent of cases from the anterior part of the nasal septum, and can therefore usually be controlled by local pressure. The child should sit erect, blow the nose to remove blood clots, and the doctor (or mother) then holds the nose for at least 10 full minutes, *not* releasing pressure every minute or two in order to determine whether bleeding is continuing. The aim is to apply pressure for sufficiently long for the normal clotting time to permit bleeding to cease. The fingers should be so placed that the whole of the anterior part of the nasal septum is compressed, the direction of the fingers being from the eyes to the mouth.

If the above method fails, one would insert a cotton wool pledget soaked in 1 in 1,000 adrenaline, but it would be unwise to leave it in place, for it might be inhaled.

If the nose is still bleeding, the child should be referred to hospital.

ERB'S PALSY

There is no need to splint the baby. Provided that the nerve root has not been torn, Erb's palsy is a self-righting condition not requiring treatment. It may or may not be of value to see that the wrist and elbow are put through a full range of movements several times a day.

Reference

ADLER J.B. & PATTERSON R. (1967) Erb's palsy. Long term results of treatment in 88 cases. *J. Bone and Joint Surgery*, **49**A, 1052.

ERYTHEMA NODOSUM

There is no specific treatment. Erythema nodosum used to be due mainly to tuberculosis, and even now it is essential to eliminate that infection. Hence any child with erythema nodosum should be referred to a paediatrician for investigation.

The usual cause of erythema nodosum is now a streptococcal infection, and this should be treated. There are other rare causes which need not be considered here; they include sulphonamides, sarcoidosis and some unusual infections.

There is nothing to be achieved by giving medicine for the erythema nodosum *per se*, though the cause should be treated. It is extremely doubtful whether there is anything to be gained by bed rest, unless there is pain which is relieved by keeping the legs elevated. This can be achieved better in a chair without enforcing bed rest.

EYE (Dilatation of the pupil for ophthalmoscopy)

I suggest that either of the following be used for routine use, being quicker acting and safer than homatropine:
Cyclopentolate (Cyclogyl, Mydrilate);
Tropicamide (Mydriacyl).

169

EYE, FOREIGN BODY IN

If the foreign body is lying on the upper or lower eyelid, removal is simple. If it lies on the cornea, it is wise to attempt to wash it out or to remove it with moistened cotton wool on an applicator. If the foreign body is metallic, the child should be referred forthwith to hospital for radiological examination and expert treatment.

FACIAL PALSY

By far the commonest cause of acute facial palsy of the lower motor neurone type is the so-called Bell's palsy, but there are other causes, such as poliomyelitis, herpes of the external auditory canal and mastoid infection. It would be wise to refer the child with Bell's palsy to a specialist for establishment of the diagnosis and prognosis; he may do this by estimating the nerve excitability (Salam & Elyahky 1968), though it is known that at least 90 per cent of children recover spontaneously.

The cornea should be protected by a drop of mineral oil at bedtime, and by an eye pad by day. It is doubtful whether nicotinic acid (50 mg. twice a day for five days) is of value. Tetracosactrin (Synacthen), or prednisolone 50 mg. per day for five days, may possibly speed recovery if given in the first five days, but it is difficult to prove this; the corticosteroids should not be given for more than five days, if at all. Taverner, Kemble & Cohen (1967) advocated the use of ACTH gel for adults, with decompression of the nerve trunk at the site of the lesion if the ACTH does not halt progressive loss of nerve excitability; but this probably applies to adults only, in whom the prognosis is not so good as in children.

The use of heat, massage, galvanic stimulation, strapping the face and cervical sympathetic block are not of value. In fact it is probable that in the case of children, no treatment is necessary or useful (except protection of the eye).

Facial palsy associated with acute otitis media usually clears up with proper treatment of the otitis media. If facial palsy occurs in chronic ear disease, referral to an ENT surgeon is essential, so that the appropriate operation can be performed.

If delayed facial palsy occurs after a head injury, a surgical opinion should be sought immediately, for an operation may be necessary to decompress the nerve.

References

ANON. (1968) Treatment for facial palsy. *Drug and Therapeutics Bulletin*, 6, 25.
SALAM E.A. & ELYAHKY W.S. (1968) Evaluation of prognosis and treatment in Bell's Palsy in children. *Acta Paediat. Scand.* 57, 468.
TAVERNER D., KEMBLE F. & COHEN S.B. (1967) *Brit. Med. J.* 4, 581.

FEVER

The family doctor is so accustomed to treating the child with a raised temperature, that it would be superfluous to discuss the matter. The treatment must depend on the cause.

The only two points which seem to be worth making are the following. The small child is unlikely to demand sufficient fluid; hence he should be persuaded to drink an adequate amount, by offering him pleasant-tasting drinks. But it may be unwise to give the infant or toddler sugary drinks, because they increase the solute load. In a Children's Hospital one commonly sees severe dehydration and even uraemia in small children, especially mentally defective ones, who have taken insufficient fluid when suffering from a simple respiratory infection.

The only other point concerns bed rest (see p. 13). There is no virtue in confining a child to bed because of fever due to a common infection, if he would prefer to be sitting up in a chair in a warm room.

FLAT FOOT

The diagnosis of flat foot as a cause of symptoms in a child is almost invariably wrong. In fact, treatment of so-called flat foot in a child is hardly ever necessary. Corrective shoes are not required.

The normal foot of the infant rarely has a distinct longitudinal arch and never a transverse one. Pads of fat give the impression of a flat foot. If a child stands on his toes, a definite longitudinal arch usually appears; and if in addition the child will stand on his heels with the front of the feet off the floor, it is almost certain that the foot is normal.

As Sharrard wrote (1964) the flat foot 'gives rise to a tremendous amount of anxiety in parents, school teachers and school clinic doctors. The only person who is seldom troubled at all is the child. To have a foot that looks flat is quite normal at the age of 1 year. Practically all children walk on the inner sides of their feet when they first start to walk.' 'It has recently been appreciated that only a very small proportion, less than 5 per cent of flat footed children continue to be flat footed indefinitely.' Sharrard wrote that if a child has a marked flat foot and markedly wears down the inner sides of the heel, the inner side of the heel should be built up by $\frac{3}{16}$ inch; this will not normally be necessary after the age of 9 or 10. Otherwise no treatment is needed.

If a child continues to complain of painful feet, in spite of satisfactory shoes, the advice of an orthopaedic expert should be sought.

Reference

Sharrard W.J.W. in Illingworth R.S. (1964) *The Normal School Child.* London, Heinemann.

FOREIGN BODY SWALLOWED

When a child swallows a foreign body, the action to be taken must depend on the nature of the object swallowed. The most important treatment usually consists of allaying parental anxiety. If the child is treated at home, there is no place for the use of purgatives or any other medicine. In many cases the child will be referred to hospital so that radiological examination will enable the doctor to assure the parents that the object has been passed. Occasionally an object such as a large hair grip becomes lodged in the intestine and has to be removed surgically.

FUNNEL CHEST (Pectus Excavatum)

In the majority of cases, no treatment is required. It is only the more severe funnel chest which can lead to respiratory embarrassment, and it is for these, and for cosmetic reasons, that a paediatric surgeon may operate. Polgar & Koop (1963) carried out pulmonary studies in 12 affected children and found that the results were normal in all; they concluded that there was no indication for surgical intervention. Others have found a gradual loss of pulmonary function after repeated respiratory infections, with the eventual development of emphysema, and consider that operation should be performed by the age of 8–12 years while the rib cage is still elastic.

It would be wise to refer children with marked funnel chest to a paediatric surgeon for advice.

References

BAY V., FARTHMANN E. & NAEGELE U. (1970) Unoperated funnel chest in middle and advanced age: evaluation of indications for operation. *J. Ped. Surgery*, 5, 606.

JENSEN N.K., SCHMIDT W.R., GARAMELLA J.J. & LYNCH M.F. (1970) Pectus Excavatum. The how, when and why of surgical correction. *J. Ped. Surgery*, 5, 4.

POLGAR G. & KOOP C.F. (1963) Pulmonary function in pectus excavatum. *Pediatrics*, 32, 209.

GINGIVITIS

Gingivitis is likely to be due to phenytoin, failure to clean the teeth, malocclusion, mouthbreathing, vitamin deficiency or blood diseases. It can often be prevented by proper care of the teeth, with the advice of the Child Welfare Clinic doctor, the School Medical Officer and the family doctor.

Gingivitis is almost usual in children being treated by phenytoin. It is not related to the dosage of the drug. Simple mouthwashes may be used, but no other treatment is helpful. It subsides a few months after discontinuing the drug.

The treatment of the other conditions depends on the cause.

GOITRE

A child with a goitre should be referred to a consultant for establishment of the nature of the thyroid enlargement and for advice about treatment. Sporadic goitre in a child is treated by thyroxin 0·025–0·05 mg. per day, in order to reduce the thyroid-stimulating action of the pituitary gland. It will be discontinued as soon as the thyroid swelling has subsided.

GROWING PAINS

As we do not understand the cause of so-called growing pains, it is difficult to advise about treatment. It is certain that the term 'growing pains' is a bad one, for they do not occur especially at the period of maximum growth; they are better termed 'limb pains'. As Apley & MacKeith (1962) put it, 'bodily growth is not painful, though emotional growth may well be'. Apley regarded the condition as similar to that of non-organic recurrent abdominal pain and headaches in children, and considered that they were commonly of psychological origin. They found that there was frequently a family history of the same complaint. Rightly or wrongly I have not myself been impressed by the emotional aspect of children suffering from these pains, but have no better idea as to what causes them. Nevertheless, it would be sensible to try to remove any obvious psychological factors. I would be reluctant to prescribe any sedative at night for such a chronic condition, with the exception of an aspirin for a severe case.

References

Apley J. (1959) *The Child with Abdominal Pains.* Oxford, Blackwell Scientific Publications.
Apley J. & MacKeith R. (1962) *The Child and his Symptoms.* Oxford, Blackwell Scientific Publications.

GYNAECOMASTIA

Enlargement of the breasts in an adolescent boy is normal and does not require treatment, because it subsides spontaneously in a year or two. The boy may need reassuring, but that is all. Before accepting this diagnosis, the family doctor should examine the testes, in order to satisfy himself that they are of normal size. If in doubt, he should refer the boy to a specialist for an opinion, for there are many possible causes of gynaecomastia, such as Klinefelter's syndrome.

Fat boys may appear to have breast enlargement, when in fact the appearance is merely due to fatty tissue.

HAEMOPHILIA AND CHRISTMAS DISEASE

The family doctor has the task of helping the parents to allow an affected child to live as normal a life as possible, though avoiding unnecessary and obvious sources of trauma at play. The padding of the playpen, cots, child's knees and forehead, may allow more play than if nothing is done to prevent injury. The doctor should discourage overprotection at home. It is better for the child to go to an ordinary school if possible, but he may have to go to a school for physically handicapped children.

Intramuscular injections of antibiotics and injections for the purpose of immunization should be avoided except under the advice of the haemophilia centre. I have several times seen serious bleeding, requiring transfusion, following injections of vaccines or antibiotics. The child should have his teeth examined regularly by a dentist, so that the risk of extraction followed by bleeding is avoided. A child with haemophilia should not be given aspirin, because of the risk of haemorrhage; it should be replaced by paracetamol if such a drug is required at all. All children with haemophilia should be seen regularly at the regional haemophilia centre.

Small cuts commonly do not cause trouble. They should be washed, and then a clean dressing soaked in Stypven is applied. For more severe haemorrhage, referral to hospital is urgent. The full development of serious bleeding after an injury usually takes two or three hours, and there is therefore time to send the child to the regional centre. Any child with a painful swollen joint or muscle, or with bleeding causing a swelling in the neck or mouth, or with haematuria, melaena, severe abdominal pain, or suspected bleeding in connection with an acute tonsillitis, should be referred to hospital immediately. If a wound requires stitching, the child should be sent to hospital unstitched, so that appropriate antihaemophilic treatment can first be given.

Drugs used by the specialist include cryoprecipitate, epsilon amino-caproic acid, and perhaps corticosteroids; the child may be given a blood or plasma transfusion.

The haemophilia centre gives the child a green card, which must always be carried, and always shown to the doctor or dentist who treats him.

Useful information can be obtained from the Haemophilia Society, PO Box 9, 16 Trinity Street, London SE1.

See also Medic-Alert, p. 64.

HAIR PLUCKING

Hair plucking, whether the child's own hair or the hair or wool of clothes or blankets, is a manifestation of insecurity. Any source of unhappiness at home or school should be sought. No medicine will help.

HALITOSIS

This is an unusual symptom in childhood. If it is of recent onset, it may be due to a foreign body in the nose. In other cases it may be due to Vincent's infection in the mouth and food debris in between teeth. The cause of the halitosis should be treated.

Reference

Anon. (1969) Halitosis. *Drug and Therapeutics Bulletin*, 7, 79.

HALLUX VALGUS

Hallux valgus is commonly familial. When a child has hallux valgus, the family doctor should refer him to the orthopaedic surgeon for advice. If the condition is mild, there may be nothing more to do than to attend to the shoes, making sure that the inner side of the shoe is reasonably straight. A severe hallux valgus may call for surgical treatment.

HANDEDNESS

If a child is consistently left-handed, no effort should be made to cause him to use the right hand in preference. If he is ambidextrous, which is more usual, no harm will be done by encouraging him to use the right hand, as long as there is no unpleasantness or display of anxiety about it.

HANDICAPPED CHILDREN – COUNSELLING THE PARENTS

The family doctor has an important role in guiding and encouraging the parents of handicapped children. He may be the first to suspect that a baby is abnormal, or he may be told by a midwife or health visitor that a baby is suspected of being abnormal. He may have the difficult task of breaking the news to the parents that all may not be well with a baby. It is a good general rule that one should never breathe a suspicion to the parents that a child is abnormal until one is certain, for even the slightest suspicion of an abnormality will cause the greatest anxiety in the parents. I received a telephone call from a family doctor one evening to say that there was a gravely distressed mother in his surgery. She had been told by a clinic doctor, 'Your child may be spastic, but don't worry.' She was extremely upset and went that evening to her family doctor for advice. I realized that it was essential that I should see the child next day, although there was no vacant appointment time. I found the baby to be entirely normal. I have many times been able to allay anxiety in parents who had been told that their child was mentally defective or spastic or hydrocephalic, when in fact he was normal. The family doctor's difficulty is that he cannot refer a child to a specialist without giving a reason for wanting the specialist's opinion. There should be a minimum of delay between expressing the doubts to the parents and the hospital consultation, because parents will worry so much in the intervening period.

I am sure that the mother should be told about a child's backwardness (*e.g.* mongolism) as soon as possible after the puerperium. It may be wiser not to tell her in the first few days after delivery. It is wrong to leave a mother to find out for herself. She is apt to have lingering doubts which she fears to ventilate even to her husband. Worry is prolonged, and there is everything to be said for letting the mother know the truth. I have asked numerous mothers as to when they feel they should be told the truth, and all have said unhesitatingly, 'As soon as possible.' Tizard & Grad (1962) found that only 7 of 218 mothers of defective children felt that they should have been left to find out for themselves. Failure to tell the parents leads to resentment against the doctor – and to distressing and expensive 'shopping round' for opinions.

At one time I thought that it might be wise to tell the father first. Many feel that this is undesirable, and that if possible the mother and father should be told simultaneously. I agree with this; a family doctor can tell both simultaneously, but it may be difficult or impossible for a consultant to do so, because a request that both parents should come next time will cause worry.

A family doctor is likely to feel real sympathy for the parents when he breaks the news to them. Whoever tells the parent, it is important to avoid such words as 'idiot', 'imbecile', 'mental defective', 'it's his brain', 'ineducable', and 'hopeless'. It is absolutely wrong for anyone to tell the parents that the baby or child has suffered 'brain damage' or 'birth injury', because that implies that the obstetrician, doctor or midwife caused the tragedy. The great majority of cases of mental deficiency and cerebral palsy were prenatal in origin. The fact that anoxia at birth may well have been due to an underlying brain defect, which caused both the respiratory depression and the mental deficiency, is commonly ignored. The same applies to mental deficiency following premature delivery; something may well have caused both the premature labour and the mental deficiency. It is most unfair to cast unjustified aspersions on the obstetrician or midwife. If a tragedy befalls one, it is much better that one should feel that it was unavoidable than to feel that it could have been avoided. I have seen innumerable parents distressed at being told that the child had suffered brain damage. One mother told me that 'it was brutal' to say so. I think that one should merely say that the child is backward or retarded.

The family doctor would be wise to leave as much as possible to the specialist with regard to the extent of the child's disability and therefore to the prognosis. It is often extremely difficult to give a prognosis, and the family doctor should not attempt to do this. The parents naturally want to know whether the child will learn to walk, talk, go to school and earn his living. It is wise to leave this to the specialist to discuss. It can be said, however, that if a child has an IQ score (or developmental quotient) of over 50, and has no additional handicap in the way of cerebral palsy, deafness or blindness, he will probably be able to earn his living.

It is sensible to emphasize the child's assets rather than his disabilities, and to discuss how the parents can live a reasonably normal life, rather than to concentrate on the difficulties which they will experience.

It is equally or even more unwise for the family doctor to give genetic advice, but he may certainly be called on to advise about birth control. The parents must know what the chances are that another child will be affected, but this is a matter for the expert. It may well be necessary to carry out numerous investigations before it is possible to express a reasonably accurate opinion about the genetic risk.

The family doctor must be conversant with the common attitudes of parents of handicapped children. When first told, they may feel resentment against the doctor and quite unjustifiably say that he was brusque or unkind. They are apt to feel guilt because of the child's handicap – guilt for a variety of reasons, such as the use of contraceptives (if Catholic), deliberately delaying conception, the amount of exercise taken during pregnancy, or efforts to end the pregnancy. They are liable to try to find someone or something to blame for the tragedy. They should be assured that the handicap is no fault of theirs or of anyone else. For this reason it is unwise to ask the parents whether anyone among their distant relatives has been affected. If the father (or his mother) is able to think of some distant relative who was backward, had fits or was spastic, he may blame himself and his wife will blame him; if the mother can think of anyone on her side who was affected, a similar thing happens. It is in fact impossible to relate the child's backwardness to the same problem in some distant relative.

The parents will certainly feel hurt pride, disappointment and often a difficulty in facing their neighbours or relatives.

An almost universal attitude is failure to accept the diagnosis. It is extremely common for parents to tell one that their seriously defective child has a 'fantastic memory', or is 'very intelligent'. They are unable to relate his achievements to an average child of the same age. When the child is older, this attitude is apt to bring the parents into conflict with the education authorities, on the grounds that the child should be in an ordinary school when he is attending a school for educationally subnormal (ESN) children, or in an ESN school when he attends a training centre.

The family doctor must be prepared to see the parents develop a pathological attachment to the child, refusing to let anyone else look after him even for an hour, worrying about the most trivial symptoms which they would ignore in a normal child, and devoting all their time and love and money to him at the cost of their normal children. The parents are almost certain to show favouritism to the handicapped child and as a result cause the other children to feel jealous. This pathological attachment may have a disastrous effect on the family and on domestic harmony. The father may himself feel jealous because of his wife's intense devotion to the child. It is a most difficult attitude to deal with, but the family doctor can at least try to point out the dangers of the attitude and its consequences.

The family doctor is in a good position to guide the parents about the child's management. The child must be taught independence, whereas it is the natural reaction of the parents of a handicapped child to do everything for him, instead of teaching him to look after himself. The doctor may guide the parents about the extremely difficult matter of teaching discipline. He guides them about the prevention of obesity if the child is inactive, because this will make it so much more difficult for the parents to look after him. He will guide them about the child's appetite, about his sleep and many other aspects of management.

The parents need advice about giving the child love and security. The mentally subnormal child is likely to cling to his mother and demand her presence and love long after the normal child has acquired a measure of independence from the mother. Such love and security must not be denied.

The mentally subnormal child and most children with cerebral palsy are late in learning to speak. There is no point in referring such a child to a hospital for speech therapy until he is speaking (but speaking indistinctly), because a speech therapist cannot make a child speak until he is ready for it. Nevertheless, if a child is late in talking it is always as well to have his hearing checked. A mentally subnormal child is more likely to have a hearing defect than a mentally normal child. It is most important that the parents should not try to make the child speak by refusing to respond to him unless he speaks. Children fail to speak because they cannot speak, and attempts to make them speak in this way are likely to cause serious behaviour problems because they cannot make their wants known.

There is a high incidence of fits in mentally subnormal children and an even higher incidence in those with cerebral palsy. It is usually impossible to stop fits in such children, but one may be able to reduce their frequency and severity. A specialist should be consulted about this.

The family doctor may be asked to advise about institutional care. This is a difficult matter which must ultimately be decided by the parents, but the doctor has to be able to discuss the pros and cons. He must know about the difficulty of arranging care in an institution, and the long years of waiting for a place. The doctor's advice will depend on the type and severity of the mental handicap, the child's aggressiveness and behaviour, the age and physical fitness of the parents, the effect on the siblings and the question of whether the defective child is preventing a further pregnancy or the adoption of a normal child. It is wrong to argue that mongols are placid and easy to manage; they are no different from other defective children of the same level of intelligence. The doctor will consider the financial, emotional and physical stresses caused by the defective child. He must be on the alert for deteriorating marital relationships. It is difficult for the father when his wife devotes her whole life to the handicapped child; marital relationships may suffer; he is apt to feel jealous of the child. The family doctor is in a good position to see whether the normal siblings are suffering as a result of the presence of the handicapped child in the home. They may suffer because of the deteriorating marital relationships of their parents, or because of the favouritism shown to the defective child, or because of the financial and physical burden and their mother's constant fatigue and resulting bad temper. The doctor may immediately see all this, while the parents are blind to it.

It should be remembered that the affected child does not benefit from being placed in an institution; it is the parents and the family who benefit. There can be little argument that it is better for the mentally defective child to be in his own home; his IQ will fall when he is placed in an institution, while parents in a good home will help him to achieve the best of which he is capable. He needs the love and security of a good home; yet one has to consider the whole family, and not just one child. The family doctor has to look at the problem from all sides – and advise the parents accordingly. He will call regularly in the early days, though as the child grows older, the intervals will be longer.

It is extremely difficult in this country for parents of a defective child such as a mongol to place the child at birth, though in the United States the practice is common. Many feel that parents who do this may have a feeling of guilt and of fear that a mistaken assessment has been made, and that it is better for parents to look after a defective child as long as they can before placing him in an institution. It is a matter which must depend on a variety of circumstances, including the personality of the parents.

The parents should be encouraged to join a parents' association – the National Society for Mentally Handicapped Children, 86 Newman Street, London W1.

The following is a list of books which the family doctor may safely recommend to the parents of a defective child:

The Subnormal Child at Home by F.J. Schonell, J.A. Richardson and T.S. McConnel. 1958. Macmillan, London.

Caring for Intellectually Handicapped Children by R. Winterbourne. New Zealand Council for Educational Research, Wellington.

Mentally Handicapped Children by National Association for Mental Health, 39 Queen Anne Street, London W1.

The Child Who Never Grew by P. Buck. 1951. Methuen, London.

Children Who Never Go to School National Association for Mental Health, 39 Queen Anne Street, London W1.

Simple Beginnings in the Training of Mentally Defective Children by M. McDowell. National Association for Mental Health, 39 Queen Anne Street, London W1.

The Retarded Child by H. Loewy. 1951. Staples Press Ltd, London.

You and Your Retarded Child by S. Kirk. 1955. Macmillan, New York.

The following address may be useful: The Elizabeth FitzRoy Home for the Handicapped Trust, Whitegates, Liss, Hampshire.

References

ILLINGWORTH R.S. (1962) Some points about the guidance of parents of mentally subnormal children. *J. Mental Subnormality*, 8, 3.

TIZARD J. & GRAD J.C. (1961) *The Mentally Handicapped and their Families*. Oxford, Oxford University Press.

HARE LIP

There is some difference of opinion among surgeons as to the age at which a hare lip should be operated upon. Many prefer to operate on the infant when he is 2–3 months old.

HAY FEVER

The treatment of hay fever is unsatisfactory. General measures include the reduction of dust in the bedroom, along the lines suggested under the section on asthma. It has been suggested that the child's bed should be covered with a plastic sheet which is removed at bedtime. There should be no flowers in the bedroom. The window must be kept shut.

Antihistamines may help some children, but most of them cause drowsiness. This may be convenient at night, but is a nuisance during the day. It is thought that phenindamine (Thephorin) and perhaps chlorpheniramine (Piriton) are less likely to cause drowsiness than other drugs. Promethazine (Phenergan) is suitable for the night, because it tends to cause drowsiness. I have no experience of brompheniramine maleate elixir which has been advocated for the purpose. Disodium cromoglycate is said to be of value for preventing symptoms.

For itching of the eyes, corticosteroid eye drops are available. Some have recommended betamethazone disodium phosphate 0·1 per cent drops for the purpose. A preparation of which I have no experience is the otrivine-antistin eye drops (Ciba) (1–2 drops b.d.) (Xylometazoline hydrochloride and antazoline sulphate). If a child has rubbed the eyes so much that there is oedema of the conjunctiva, a drop or two of 1 in 4,000 adrenaline gives immediate relief.

For nasal congestion I do not advise nose drops because they may damage the nasal cilia. I have not found corticosteroid snuff of value, and one must remember that it will be absorbed. Some advocate the wearing of dark spectacles when outside in the sun.

I have discussed the role of hyposensitization on p. 88.

Preparations

Chlorpheniramine (NF) is cheaper than the proprietary equivalent Piriton.

Tablets 4 mg.   Dose up to 1 year   2·5 ml. b.d.
Syrup 2 mg. in 5 ml.   1–5 years   2·5–5·0 ml. b.d.
                       6–12 years   4 mg. t.d.

Brompheniramine maleate (Dimotane)
4 mg. tablets; elixir 2 mg. in 5 ml.
Age 2–4 years 5 ml. t.d.

Phenindamine (Theophorin) 25 mg. tablets.
Older child 1 tablet b.d. or t.d.

References

ANON. (1967) Adrenaline eye drops. *Drug and Therapeutics Bulletin*, **5**, 99.

HOLOPAINEN E., BACKMAN A. & SALO O.P. (1971) Effect of disodium cromoglycate on seasonal allergic rhinitis. *Lancet*, **1**, 55.

MACAULAY D.B. (1967) The treatment of hayfever. *Prescribers' Journal*, **7**, 19.

HEADACHE

See *Migraine*.

HEAD BANGING

Head banging is an annoying habit seen mainly between the ages of 9 months and 4 years. The child takes pleasure in banging his head against the end of the bed, or on the floor, or against the wall, hard chairs or the table. It is commonly associated with insecurity – unkindness in the home, excessive strictness, domestic friction, or perhaps jealousy. The family doctor, knowing the family, is in a better position than anyone to determine the cause of the problem. Treatment must depend on the cause. Medicines are not indicated. Because head banging may be followed by cataract formation, expert advice should be sought.

Reference

SPALTER H.F., BEMPORAD J.R. & SOURS J.A. (1970) Cataracts following head banging. *Arch. Ophthalmol.* **83**, 182.

HEAD INJURY

If there is any possibility of concussion or of fractured skull, as evidenced by retrograde amnesia, vomiting, convulsion or confusion after an accident, escape of blood from the ear or CSF rhinorrhoea, the child should be sent to hospital immediately. A fracture may occur without any of these symptoms, and when in doubt the family doctor will send the child to hospital for X-ray.

If the child is not admitted, it is important that the parents should watch for and immediately report increasing drowsiness, inability to arouse the child, increasing headache, vomiting, undue irritability, incessant crying or loss of interest in toys and play. If a child develops any of these symptoms after a head injury, he should be sent to hospital immediately.

CONGENITAL HEART DISEASE

A child with congenital heart disease will be under the supervision of a paediatrician or paediatric cardiologist, who will seek the advice of a cardiothoracic surgeon about the possibility of surgical treatment. But in the intervals between visits to the paediatrician, the family doctor will be concerned with the care of the infant in an illness. If the infant develops what appears to be bronchopneumonia, he should refer the child to the hospital immediately, because he may have heart failure which requires digitalization. This must be carried out by the expert, who may refer the child back to the family doctor on a maintenance dose. The maintenance dose of dictoxin is usually 0·005 to 0·01 mg./kg./day. The family doctor needs to be conversant with the signs of overdosage – reduced urinary output, vomiting, loss of appetite, coupling of the beats or bradycardia.

As far as possible the child should be treated as a normal child, without any effort to restrict his exercise. He should be left to regulate the exercise himself, deciding for himself how much he can do. Overprotection must be avoided.

HEIGHT, EXCESSIVE

When a parent is abnormally tall, and a girl is showing signs of excessive height, the doctor may be asked whether anything can be done to retard growth. Attempts have been made to achieve this; Whitelaw & Foster (1962) attempted to stop excessive growth by intermittent injections of estradiol valerate and 17 hydroxyprogesterone caproate, and claimed some success. Wettenhall & Roche (1965) were less optimistic; they prescribed stilboestrol 3 mg./day until growth ceased. The treatment is not without risk, as was pointed out in Leading Articles in the *Lancet* and the *British Medical Journal* (1963). I personally feel doubtful whether the treatment is justifiable.

References

ANON. (1963) Drugs for altering the growth of children (leading article). *Brit. Med. J.* 1, 1035.

ANON. (1963) The tall girl (leading article). *Lancet*, 1, 368.

WETTENHALL H.N.B. & ROCHE A.F. (1965) Tall girls. Assessment and management. *Australian Paediat. J.* 1, 210.

WHITELAW, M.J. & FOSTER T.N. (1962) Treatment of excessive height in girls. *J. Pediat.* 61, 566.

HEPATITIS, INFECTIVE

If a child has been exposed to infective hepatitis, he can be protected if thought necessary by injection of 0·04 mg./kg. of gammaglobulin intramuscularly as long as it is given within a week of exposure. It protects for about three months. If a child is to be taken to a country abroad where infective hepatitis is prevalent, a dose of 0·06–0·12 mg./kg. of gammaglobulin should prevent the disease. A review in the *Drug and Therapeutics Bulletin* (1970) advocated 250 mg. intramuscularly for a child under 10 years, and 500 mg. over that age. It gives protection for six months.

There is no specific treatment for the disease, and no medicine is necessary. The general principles of rest have been discussed elsewhere.

As a result of experience in the treatment of many hundreds of cases of infective hepatitis in the Middle East, I concluded that rest was essential in that condition – though I cannot say that the patients would not have fared equally well if they had been allowed to rest in the ward without staying in bed. I saw innumerable officers and soldiers in whom jaundice had continued for a prolonged period of ambulant activity, but which settled promptly on rest. Capps & Barker (1947) after a controlled study of 8,000 cases in the Middle East, considered that bed rest was essential, and that activity predisposed to relapse. Chalmers (1955), however, in a carefully controlled study of an outbreak in Korea, studied 126 soldiers on complete rest and 127 allowed ordinary ward activity, and found no difference in the results. Repsher & Freebern (1969) went further, and gave one group of 199 patients vigorous exercise and compared the results with those in 199 controls – finding no difference at all. The leading article following this paper pointed out that the cases were not selected by random sampling, there was a possibility of bias in the study, the patients were all young men, and there was no record of those cases which were excluded or withdrawn from the study. I personally would prefer that a patient of mine with infective hepatitis should rest, not necessarily in bed, but that ordinary activity should not be allowed. I fully recognize that it is a matter of opinion. Furthermore, if the child is ill, or if the jaundice is not clearing within a fortnight, I would recommend that he should be sent to hospital; it is a potentially serious disease for which good nursing and specialist treatment may be required.

There is no need to restrict the fat in the diet, unless the child himself feels that he cannot take fat. A normal diet should otherwise be given.

187

The disease is infectious from sixteen days before the jaundice begins to eight days after the appearance of the jaundice.

References

ANON. (1970) Infectious hepatitis; protection by immunoglobulin. *Drug and Therapeutics Bulletin*, 8, 33.

CAPPS R.B. & BARKER M.H. (1947) Management of infective hepatitis. *Ann. Int. Med* 26, 405.

CHALMERS J.T. (1955) The treatment of acute infectious hepatitis. *J. Clin. Invest.* 34 1163.

REPSHER L.H. & FREEBERN R.K. (1969) Effects of early and vigorous exercise on recovery from infectious hepatitis. *New Engl. J. Med.* 281, 1393. (See also leading article. p. 1421.)

SILVERBERG M., WHERETT B., WORDEN E. & NEUMANN P.Z. (1969) An evaluation of rest and low fat diets in the management of acute infective hepatitis. *J. Pediat.* 74, 260.

HERNIA

An inguinal hernia should be operated upon as soon as it is diagnosed, because there is an ever-present risk of strangulation. The younger the child, the greater the risk of strangulation, and so the greater the need for an early operation.

An umbilical hernia normally cures itself. Strangulation is extremely rare. There is no need to apply strapping to the hernia; the strapping is apt to irritate the skin and it achieves nothing. There is evidence that strapping may actually retard healing. An umbilical hernia may cure itself even as late as 4 or 5 years of age. Until then the question of surgical treatment does not arise.

It is said that a supra-umbilical hernia, which does not involve the umbilicus, will not cure itself and requires operation. There is virtually no danger of strangulation, and operation, though eventually necessary, is not a matter of urgency.

Reference

WALKER S.H. (1967) The natural history of umbilical hernia. *Clinical Pediatrics*, 6, 29.

HERPES

Herpes may be a serious generalized infection in a newborn baby, and any adult with herpes on the lip ('cold sores') should be kept away from such a baby.

No special treatment is required for herpes labialis, for it is a self-limiting condition. I do not think that the use of idoxuridine ointment is justified.

Herpetic stomatitis is a self-limiting condition, lasting about ten days, but parents expect some treatment, because it is such an unpleasant condition for the child. The lesions may be painted with dequalinium chloride paint (Dequadin). Cold drinks, ice creams and drinks taken through a straw give the child some comfort.

Herpatic infection of the eye will be treated by the ophthalmologist – probably with idoxuridine.

HICCOUGH

I have never found it necessary to prescribe treatment for hiccough in a child. It is said that chlorpromazine is the most effective drug if a drug has to be used.

Chlorpromazine (Largactil) can be given as syrup 25 mg. in 5 ml., or as tablets of 10 mg., 25 mg., or 50 mg. The dose at ages between 2 weeks and 1 year is 1 mg./kilo/t.d.

HIP, TRANSIENT SYNOVITIS (Irritable hip)

The child who develops a limp due to the hip must be referred to the orthopaedic specialist. If the child has the common 'transient synovitis of hip', he will be kept in bed for one or two weeks or until his symptoms have subsided, but he will be followed up in case he turns out to have Perthes' disease.

HODGKIN'S DISEASE

The child with Hodgkin's disease will be under the care of a consultant. The treatment is likely to include vincristine, cyclophosphamide, procarbazine, corticosteroids or nitrogen mustard, and may include radiotherapy.

Signs of deterioration in the child's condition include pallor, purpura, abdominal pain, fever, cough or stridor, with increasing lassitude.

See also *Death and Dying* p. 138.

HUMERUS, FRACTURED, IN THE NEWBORN

This is treated as a first-aid measure by bandaging the arm across the chest, with the elbow bent. Orthopaedic advice is then sought.

HYDROCEPHALUS

A child with suspected hydrocephalus should be referred to a paediatric surgeon in order that the diagnosis may be established and a suitable shunt operation performed. Untreated, optic atrophy, blindness and spasticity are liable to develop, the head undergoes unsightly enlargement, and the mental development is likely to suffer. There can be little excuse for leaving a child with moderate or severe hydrocephalus (without spina bifida) untreated.

HYDROCOELE

In the first year of life a hydrocoele is left to cure itself. If it has not cured itself by the age of 12 months or so, it is nearly always associated with a hernia, and surgery is required.

HYPERTRICHOSIS

Hypertrichosis may be due to phenytoin, corticosteroids or diazoxide. It occurs in any severe wasting disease, Cushing's syndrome, porphyria and lipodystrophy.

The treatment is that of the cause.

HYPOSPADIAS

The decision as to the need for operation depends on the direction of the stream of urine. If the flow is not in the normal forward direction, but the urine leaks from the under surface of the penis on to the floor, down the child's legs or on to his shoes, operation is needed. This is usually done at the age of 3 or 4 years. It is desirable for psychological reasons that the operation should be performed before the child starts school.

It is important that the diagnosis should be verified immediately. It is easy to make the mistake of diagnosing hypospadias when the child is a girl with adrenocortical hyperplasia with resulting virilization. A buccal smear clinches the diagnosis.

ICHTHYOSIS

A new treatment worth trying is Calnurid, a urea cream. It is applied after a bath, left on five minutes, and the excess is then wiped off. Boots E.45 is also useful.

Reference

ANON. (1971) Calnurid, a urea cream for the skin. *Drug and Therapeutics Bulletin*, 9, 29.

IMPETIGO

There are differences of opinion about the treatment of impetigo – probably because so many different treatments are effective. I suggest that the average small area of impetigo should be treated by neomycin – bacitracin cream, or by chlorhexidine lotion, without attempting to remove the scabs. As the treatment is not required for more than a few days, the risk of skin sensitization is minimal. If there is underlying scabies or pediculosis, it should be treated. For more severe or extensive impetigo, I would clean the skin and affected area with chlorhexidine lotion, and give an antibiotic such as cloxacillin or erythromycin by mouth. Some would soak large firm crusts off with warm water, liquid paraffin or emplastrum plumbi and soft paraffin, equal parts, left on for 24 hours; but I doubt whether such treatment is necessary. In a severe case it is wise to take a swab before treating in order to determine the sensitivities of the organism.

An American study (Dillon 1970) of 531 children, found that the most effective treatment was benzathine penicillin G intramuscularly; it was more effective than topical bacitracin ointment. The child should be kept off school until the impetigo has been cured. If other members of the family have impetigo, they should also be treated.

Streptococcal skin infections are an important cause of nephritis. It is rational to treat them promptly with an antibiotic with the intention of preventing nephritis.

Reference

DILLON H.C. (1970) The treatment of streptococcal skin infections. *J. Pediat.* **76**, 676.

INDIGESTION

Virtually all children referred to me with the diagnosis of 'indigestion' or 'excessive wind' are toddlers with sleep refusal due to mismanagement (see *Sleep Refusal* p. 241). There is no indigestion or excessive wind.

The possibility that a child has a peptic ulcer should not be forgotten.

If in doubt, the family doctor should refer the child to a paediatrician for an opinion and, if necessary, investigation.

If any child has excessive wind, the cause of the air-swallowing should be sought, for all 'wind' is due to swallowed air .

INFLUENZA

Influenza being a virus infection, no antibiotic is available for its treatment. It is useless to prescribe penicillin or other antibiotic. Neither is there any indication for a cough medicine. It is a self-limiting infection and no medicine is indicated.

INTERTRIGO

The moist parts should be kept dry. If there is oozing, a wet dressing of calamine lotion or lotio aluminium acetate is used at first, or 3 per cent iodochlorhydroxyquinolone (Vioform). Equal parts of talc and zinc oxide are then applied four times a day to keep the part dry. 1 per cent hydrocortisone ointment may be tried if the intertrigo has not been cleared by the above method.

JAUNDICE

See *Hepatitis*.

Neonatal jaundice

The treatment depends on the cause. *Jaundice on the first day must be regarded as haemolytic disease until proved otherwise, and it is imperative that the infant should be referred immediately to the hospital for replacement transfusion if the diagnosis is confirmed.*

Jaundice on the third day is physiological until proved otherwise, and no treatment is required. If jaundice persists more than three or four days, the infant should be referred to hospital for establishment of the diagnosis.

JEALOUSY

If a child is jealous, it is because he feels that he is not loved as much as he would like, or because he has lost his feeling of importance. It may arise because of the new baby, but is often caused by favouritism or comparisons. It shows itself by one of the manifestations of insecurity – bedwetting, nightmares, nailbiting or any of many behaviour problems; diagnosis may be difficult, but it may be obvious – as when the child repeatedly hits the baby on the head or cries when his mother picks the baby up.

It is vital that the mother should not punish the child, for punishment will inevitably make him all the more convinced that he has lost his mother's love. It would be futile and harmful to treat the symptoms; it is essential to treat the cause, the feeling of loss of love, security and importance. He needs above all to be given extra love and to be made to feel more important.

In spite of the wisest of management some children remain jealous. Such jealousy is often an inherited characteristic – the mother or father showing the same feature.

The family doctor has an important part to play in helping parents with the problem of jealousy.

KNOCK-KNEE

It is surprising to some that a child who at 9 or 12 months was thought to have bow legs is at the age of 2 or 3 thought to have knock-knee.

The great majority of children cure themselves of knock-knee by the age of 6. It is normal for a toddler to have a gap of 2–3 inches between the malleoli when the knees are in contact. No operation will be carried out before the child is 8, and operation will be rare indeed. No treatment is required provided that there is no abnormal weight-bearing, as shown by abnormal shoe wear, and that there is no obvious organic disease. In either case, expert orthopaedic help should be sought, and an alteration to the shoe may be required.

Knock-knee in older children, commencing at the age of 7 or 8, is a progressive condition; a stapling operation may be needed at the age of 11 or 12 years, and perhaps an osteotomy later. There are other rare conditions associated with knock-knee, and if in doubt, the orthopaedic surgeon should be asked for his opinion.

Reference

FARRIER C.D. & LLOYD ROBERTS G.C. (1969) The natural history of idiopathic knock knee. *Practitioner*, 203, 789.

LABIAL ADHESIONS

Labial adhesions in the newborn can usually be separated by the application of 0·01 per cent dienoestrol cream to the point of adhesion. The labia usually fall apart in 10–14 days.

An alternative is to separate the adhesions by a probe, followed by the application of vaseline to the parts separated.

LARYNGOTRACHEOBRONCHITIS: ACUTE LARYNGEAL STRIDOR

If I were in General Practice again, few if any conditions would cause me more anxiety than laryngotracheobronchitis, gastroenteritis or acute abdominal pain in a young child. The difficulty is to decide at what stage the child should be sent to hospital. I advise that a pre-school child (and possibly an older child) who develops stridor should be sent to hospital immediately, for the risk of looking after him at home is too great. Furthermore, unless there is an obvious infection, there is always the possibility that the child has inhaled a foreign body.

The child with acute laryngitis may rapidly develop respiratory obstruction and urgently need a tracheostomy. It follows that if a child with acute laryngitis is to be looked after in the home, he must be seen repeatedly and frequently until one is sure that he is improving. It is not enough to see the child in the morning and then see him next day. The child with epiglottitis, which is commonly due to Haemophilus Influenzae, is particularly apt to develop obstruction of the airway. If a child's acute stridor is tending to worsen, and certainly if there is any indrawing of the lower part of the chest, or if the respiratory efforts are beginning to tire him, he should be sent to hospital without delay. An attempt to view the larynx by means of a laryngoscope might well precipitate obstruction.

The child would be treated at home with steam (*e.g.* in a bathroom). Dry oxygen tends to dry the thick mucus and should be avoided. His anxiety may be relieved by chloral. He should be persuaded to take abundant fluid – an important part of treatment. Ampicillin may be prescribed in case the infection may be due to Haemophilus Influenzae, but other antibiotics are of doubtful value.

LEAD POISONING

The treatment of lead poisoning will be in the hands of an expert. Drugs used are likely to be dimercaprol (BAL) and sodium calcium edetate (EDTA), or penicillamine.

LEFT-HANDEDNESS

See *Handedness* p. 177.

LEUKAEMIA

The treatment of leukaemia will be in the hands of a paediatrician or paediatric haematologist or both. It is likely to consist of cyclical treatment with corticosteroids, 6 mercaptopurine, methotrexate, vincristine, and perhaps asparaginase and cytosine arabinoside.

Signs of unsatisfactory progress include progressive lassitude, pallor, fever, stomatitis and purpura. Signs of neurological involvement are common; they would be manifested by headache, root pains, neck stiffness or other neurological signs, and if such involvement is suspected the child should be referred forthwith back to the hospital, in order that appropriate treatment, such as intrathecal methotrexate, can be given.

The family doctor has the difficult task of dealing with the psychological problems in the child, and trying to support the family when faced with the terrible news that the child is suffering from leukaemia.

For *Death and Dying*, see p. 138.

LYING

It is not always easy to draw the line between the normal fantasy-thinking of an imaginative 7–8-year-old child and deliberate lying; and even when the child is deliberately lying, it is difficult to draw the line between the normal and the abnormal; that which is normal at one age is not normal at another. One cannot expect a 4-year-old to be truthful; but one may hope for reasonable truthfulness from a 10-year-old. Parents need reassurance from the family doctor, for they are often worried by untruthfulness, which nevertheless may be entirely normal for the age.

The child should not have to lie because he fears punishment; he should not be punished if he tells the truth. He may lie because he fears criticism (*e.g.* about his work at school). He may lie because there is a battle of wills – his mother or father insisting on his confessing to some crime (such as accidentally breaking a window), with the result that the child, equally determined, continues his lies, and one lie leads to another.

The family doctor is in a good position to help the parents. He knows the family background. He has to determine the reason for the child's behaviour, such as worry at home or school. His parents may be over-ambitious, overdemanding, overstrict, perfectionists and unreasonable in their attitude. The child feels insecure, and his response to insecurity may be untruthfulness. Punishment will inevitably make him worse, for it will convince him all the more that he has lost his parents' love and his own feeling of importance, a feeling which is the basic cause of the trouble. The family doctor has to go into the whole management of the child and especially the parents' attitudes, if he is to give any help; and he has to convince the parents that what the child needs is not punishment, criticism and derogation, but love, encouragement, praise and security. No drugs will help.

MASTITIS, NEONATAL

No treatment is necessary. Massage of the breasts should be avoided absolutely.

MASTURBATION

As long as parents realize that almost all boys and most girls masturbate at least some time during childhood or adolescence, there will be less need for attempting treatment, because it is manifestly harmless physically, except when it is so excessive that there is actual soreness of the parts. If it is performed in public, efforts have to be made to stop it.

When the infant and small child is found to be masturbating, there are only two immediate courses of action available – either to ignore it or to distract the child by interesting him in another occupation. On no account must he be reprimanded or punished for it, for he would almost certainly continue to do it all the more.

If it is excessive, one should try to find any source of insecurity, in the way of conflict at home or school. The older child can be led to understand that it is regarded as bad manners to masturbate in public, but reprimands will not help.

The most important aspect of the treatment of masturbation is probably the allaying of parental anxieties. The parents must understand that if the child knows that they are anxious about it, it will continue. Furthermore, they must be convinced that it is harmless.

MEASLES

There is no specific treatment for measles. If the child wants to be in bed, as he will in the acute stage, he should be in bed, but he should get up as soon as he wishes. As in the case of all febrile conditions in childhood, it is important to see that he drinks sufficient fluid. An aspirin may be given for headache. There is nothing to be said for giving a cough medicine. An investigation by the College of General Practitioners showed that prophylactic antibiotics are of no value and may be harmful. If complications such as otitis media or bronchopneumonia develop, they will be treated accordingly.

For the prevention of measles, see p. 40.

Duration of infectivity

Measles is infectious from five to six days before the rash develops to five days after the temperature has become normal. Quarantine is not required. Incubation period: ten to fifteen days.

Reference

College of General Practitioners, report of a study group (1956) The complications of measles. *J. College Practitioners.*

MEATAL ULCER

A meatal ulcer is a complication of ammonia dermatitis, and is virtually confined to circumcised boys. Ammonia dermatitis is an absolute contraindication to circumcision.

The ulcer is treated by attention to the nappy rash and by the application of a local anaesthetic ointment (*e.g.* lignocaine) to the ulcer at such intervals that the pain caused by micturition is relieved.

MELAENA NEONATORUM

When a newborn baby passes blood in the stool or vomits blood, it is essential to know whether it is the mother's blood or that of the baby. If the stool or vomitus is put into water, and if necessary filtered, there will be a pink liquid; if N/5 Na OH is added, the colour will change to yellow if it is the mother's blood, but remain pink if it is the baby's blood, because foetal haemoglobin is more resistant to alkali.

If it is the mother's blood, no treatment is required; if it is the baby's blood, there is bleeding (usually from the oesophagus or duodenum) and it is essential to watch him carefully in hospital with laboratory help to ensure that blood loss is not severe. Most but not all cases are relieved by an intramuscular injection of Vitamin K (phytomenadione; trade name: Konakion) 1 mg. in 0·5 ml.

MENINGITIS

When it is suspected that a child has meningitis, it is essential that he should be referred immediately to hospital for lumbar puncture and treatment; it is a serious mistake to give an antibiotic in the home, since it may be useless for the particular infection from which the child is suffering, and it will make it difficult or impossible for the hospital doctor to recover the organism from the cerebrospinal fluid; it will then be necessary to guess the infecting organism, and the wrong antibiotic may then be given – perhaps with disastrous results.

MENORRHAGIA

A specialist would be consulted about menorrhagia. It tends to be self-limiting in an adolescent, reassurance being an important factor.

The specialist may prescribe ergometrine 0·5 mg. t.d. or norethynodrel (Enovid) 10 mg. b.d. for 2–3 weeks.

Reference

DEWHURST C.J. (1963) *Gynaecological Disorders of Infants and Children.* London, Cassell.

MIGRAINE

The treatment of migraine and allied headaches in children is unsatisfactory. Usually there is no discoverable precipitating factor, but sometimes there is a history that a long car journey, excitement or other psychological factors, fatigue, visual stress, hunger, an infection, or an article of food, precipitates attacks. If emotional factors cause attacks, it is not usually possible to do much about them, but sometimes a regular dose of phenobarbitone 30 mg. twice a day may prevent attacks. One child I saw had an attack of migraine whenever she was punished. In this case one was able to help by advice on wiser methods of exerting discipline. It is important to try to resolve any conflicts at home or school. If attacks are feared when the child is about to take an examination, a sedative may help. If attacks are brought on by television or film viewing, appropriate steps must be taken. Sun-glasses under certain circumstances may be advised. If attacks are provoked by hunger, the child should be provided with biscuits or sugar lumps to take when he is likely to be hungry and so to have an attack because of hypoglycaemia. Eye testing for refraction errors is irrelevant and therefore unnecessary.

It is worth investigating a possible dietary cause of attacks. Hanington and others (1969) have shown that tyramine-containing foods may precipitate attacks in some patients. These substances are chocolate (the worst offender), cheese (especially Cheddar and Stilton), other dairy products, fish, broad beans, Marmite and Bovril. Onions, tomatoes, cucumber, nuts and alcohol have also been incriminated. The history must be taken carefully. When I asked a mother whether any foodstuff precipitated attacks in her boy, the reply was negative. I then asked about specific foodstuffs, and when I mentioned chocolate she said that she could not answer the question about chocolate, as he never touched it.

Fortunately I asked why he would not have chocolate, and she replied that ever since he had had a bad attack after eating chocolate he had refused to have chocolate again. It would be a mistake to overemphasize the role of dietary factors, because it is probable that they are relevant in only about one in four sufferers.

The treatment of an attack is apt to be unsatisfactory because of vomiting. It is often sufficient for the child to retire to bed in a darkened room and sleep it off. It is certainly undesirable to make an unnecessary fuss about the child's attack and to transfer anxiety to him. A dose of aspirin or tab codein co may be adequate if anything has to be given. Codis tablets contain a large dose of aspirin (500 mg.) and codein 0·8 mg. It is worth trying Cafergot (ergotamine tartrate with caffeine) 1–2 tablets at the first sign of an attack. An alternative measure is to give an ergotamine tartrate spray in a medihaler at the beginning of an attack; this provides 0·36 mg. of ergotamine tartrate in one dose. An ergotamine tartrate tablet may be sucked under the tongue; it is less effective if swallowed. Ergotamine preparations must not be abused. Not more than one dose should be given in any one week, because of the fear of a sensitivity reaction, with peripheral gangrene. (Individuals vary greatly in their sensitivity to ergotamine.) Methisergide is not used in children because of the risk of retroperitoneal fibrosis.

For persistent vomiting, one may try chlorpromazine (Largactil) 10 mg. under 5 years, 10–25 mg. at the age of 5–10 years, and 25 mg. thereafter; or prochlorperazine (Stematil) but if they can be avoided they should be, because of the possible side effects.

Aspirin is cheaper than most proprietary preparations, which offer no advantages.
Tab Codein Co (BP) is cheaper than the proprietary preparations Codis or Veganin.
Paracetamol BP is cheaper than the proprietary preparation 'Panadol'.
Cafergot is composed of ergotamine tartrate 1 mg. with caffeine 100 mg.
  No specific dose is given for children.

References

ANON. (1964) The treatment of migraine. *Drug and Therapeutics Bulletin*, **2**, 57.
BILLE B. (1962) Migraine in school children. *Acta Paediatrica*, Uppsala, Suppl. 136.
FRIEDMAN A.P. & HARMS E. (1967) *Headaches in Children*. Springfield, Charles Thomas.
GRAHAM J.G. (1969) The treatment of migraine. *Prescribers' Journal*, **9**, 131.
HANINGTON E., in Smith R. (1969) *Background to Migraine*. London, Heinemann.

MONONUCLEOSIS, INFECTIOUS

There is no specific treatment for infectious mononucleosis. Antibiotics have no effect, but it is difficult to avoid the temptation of prescribing penicillin when the child has an acute tonsillitis with slough due to this virus infection. For reasons not fully understood ampicillin is especially liable to cause a severe rash, often purpuric, when taken by a child with infectious mononucleosis.

The treatment is purely symptomatic, but in fact it is hardly ever necessary to prescribe any drug. A mouthwash may be used for tonsillitis and stomatitis. There is no indication for bed rest as soon as the child is anxious to get up. Recent work has suggested that a week's course of prednisolone may give relief in a severe case.

The course is variable, but the child can usually return to school within a fortnight. I have seen children kept away from school and with restricted activity for prolonged periods without any apparent reason.

References

ANON. (1969) Corticosteroid therapy in glandular fever. *Drug and Therapeutics Bulletin*, 7, 31.

SHAPIRO S., SISKIND V., SLONE D., LEWIS G.P. & JICK H. (1969) Drug rash with ampicillin and other penicillins. *Lancet*, 2, 969.

MUMPS

There is no specific treatment for mumps. An aspirin or tab codein co may be given for severe discomfort. There is no need to keep the child in bed if he wishes to get up.

Orchitis is virtually confined to boys at or after puberty. Apart from supporting the scrotum, no treatment will help. Surgical intervention, the administration of stilboestrol or corticosteroids, has not proved to be useful.

Duration of infectivity

Mumps is infectious from two days before the swelling appears until the swelling has subsided. In the case of a unilateral swelling, the child may be infectious until it is clear that the other side is remaining unaffected. Quarantine is not required.

Incubation period: 12–26 days (especially 18 days).

MUSCULAR DYSTROPHY

There is no drug therapy for muscular dystrophy. The child should be enabled to live as normal a life as possible, without overprotection. In the later stages it is important to prevent scoliosis, for scoliosis may be severe and considerably adds to the child's handicap. An orthopaedic specialist should be consulted about a suitable spinal support.

Confinement to bed for an incidental illness should be limited to the absolute minimum, for bed rest causes rapid and severe deterioration in the child's condition.

Obesity must be prevented. There is especial danger of developing obesity, on account of the inactivity.

Parents should be encouraged to join the Muscular Dystrophy Association, 26 Borough High Street, London SE1.

Reference

Dubowitz V. (1963) Muscular dystrophy. *Brit. J. Clin. Practice*, 17, 283.

NAEVI

The 'stork bites' on the inner end of the upper eyelid, the wedge-shaped naevus on the forehead above the bridge of the nose, and the capillary naevus on the back of the neck, all disappear without treatment.

The strawberry naevus (capillary haemangioma) grows in size for up to six months, then gradually heals from the centre outwards, disappearing by 5–10 years of age. No treatment should be given, for it will disappear without a scar if left alone, while surgical or other treatment always causes scar formation. For a large naevus involving the neck and larynx, prednisone may be tried for a short period only – perhaps for two or three weeks; this treatment should not be used for the ordinary strawberry naevus, even if it covers a large part of the face. The cavernous haemangioma will also disappear if left alone. When the occasional cavernous haemangioma begins to grow unduly rapidly, the paediatric surgeon should be consulted; he may inject it with saturated saline.

The spider naevus should be left untreated; but if a girl is self-conscious about it, it can be destroyed by touching the central vessel with a diathermy needle.

The port-wine stain is best concealed by Boots' Covermark or Elizabeth Arden's Covercream. Tattooing, dermabrasion and other methods have not proved satisfactory.

Reference

Fost N.C. & Esterly N.B. (1968) Successful treatment of juvenile hemangiomas by prednisone. *J. Pediat.* **72**, 351.

NAILBITING

More than half of all children bite their nails, and it is a harmless though ugly pastime. Determined efforts to stop it are likely to make it continue as an attention-seeking device. Any discoverable cause of insecurity, such as friction at home or school, should be removed. If the child is a girl, one may appeal to her vanity by applying red varnish to the nails and trying to persuade her that she is spoiling her appearance.

Treatment is unsatisfactory.

NAPPY RASH

The commonest form of nappy rash is that caused by ammonia dermatitis. This is due to ammonia liberated by urea-splitting organisms, the bacillus ammoniagenes, proteus and pyocyaneus from the bowel acting on the urine in the nappy. Mothers note the strong smell of ammonia when the nappy is changed. It is pointless to give the baby medicine by mouth. The longer the wet nappies are in contact with the skin, the more likely it is that a rash will develop. Tightly fitting rubber or plastic pants, fitting tightly round the abdomen and thighs, encourage the development of a rash.

The first step in treating a rash is to try to ensure that the nappy is being properly washed and thoroughly rinsed, and is being changed frequently enough. My practice is to enquire about this indirectly, by asking the mother how many nappies she has. It would be difficult to manage with less than 36–48 nappies, unless one had a drying cabinet. The mother should rinse the nappies thoroughly after washing them. Some recommend that they should be rinsed in 1 in 8,000 benzalkonium chloride, with the aim of discouraging the urea-splitting organisms.

The polypropylene Marathon or Drinap nappy is useful to put next to the skin, because it allows the fluid to pass through, so that the part next to the skin remains dry.

There is no one treatment for nappy rash. Boric acid lotion or crystals must never be used, because serious and fatal poisoning may result from the absorption of the boric acid. A useful lotion to apply four or five times a day is 4 per cent tannic acid with 0·1 per cent proflavine. The various quaternary ammonium compounds are satisfactory *e.g.* benzalkonium 0·01 per cent (Drapolene, Calaxin or Roccal) in water miscible base or cream; other suitable preparations are a silicone barrier cream BPC, or zinc oxide 7·5 per cent, calamine 1·5 per cent in silicone cream. Zinc and castor oil ointment is satisfactory for a mild ammonia dermatitis. For a severe, acutely inflamed rash, $\frac{1}{2}$ per cent hydrocortisone ointment may be used *for one week only*.

A nappy rash composed of isolated vesicles is usually due to moniliasis – or at least it may be due to moniliasis secondary to ammonia dermatitis. It responds to nystatin ointment. For an acutely inflamed rash, the nystatin may be combined with hydrocortisone ointment (nystaform HC) and used for one week only.

A psoriasiform nappy rash, which as the name implies, resembles psoriasis, spreads from the nappy area to the rest of the body. It responds to Betnovate (betamethasone), or to Nystaform (nystatin with hydrocortisone) – in either case used for one week only. I have not found it necessary to use other, more expensive preparations.

A seborrhoeic or eczematous nappy rash, which is confined to the nappy area and involves the creases (*e.g.* of the groin), responds to Vioform – iodochlorhydroxyquinoline cream (Clioquinol) with hydrocortisone or Betnovate (betamethasone) used for seven days.

The reason for restricting the duration of corticosteroid treatment to a week is the risk of dermal atrophy if treatment is prolonged – and the risk of absorption.

NEGATIVISM

Mothers are often worried about the child's negativism and awkwardness; they are worried because the child who a few months ago (at the age of 6–12 months) was a charming baby with a smile for everyone, has become at 1–3 years a difficult awkward character, who can always be relied upon to do the opposite of what he is asked to do, always says No, and obstinately refuses to do as he is asked.

The family doctor can do much to reassure a mother and explain that the child's behaviour is normal. All normal children pass through a phase of negativism between 12 and about 36 months. If only the mother can understand that it is normal and take it with a sense of humour, the behaviour will cease to be a problem.

No medicine is required. Punishment is contraindicated.

NEPHRITIS, ACUTE

The child with acute nephritis is usually treated in hospital because of the danger of hypertensive encephalopathy, and because of the importance of keeping a careful record of his daily fluid intake and output. Provided, however, that the urine output is satisfactory and the blood pressure is normal, and that the family doctor can see the child daily until obvious improvement occurs, the child can be looked after at home; but if there is any elevation of blood pressure or reduction in urinary output the child should be sent to hospital.

There is no need to keep the child in bed – at least after macroscopic haematuria has disappeared. It has long been our practice to allow children with acute nephritis to be up and about the ward as soon as naked eye haematuria has ceased; and we have no evidence that it would have been harmful to have allowed them up sooner. Åkerrén & Lindgren (1955) in Sweden, and McCrory *et al.* (1958) in the United States, showed that confinement to bed did not help.

There is no indication for fluid, salt or protein restriction provided that the urinary output is satisfactory. Controlled studies have shown that protein restriction is unnecessary and undesirable.

Full recovery is usual but not invariable after acute nephritis in childhood. After the acute attack there is no question of tonsillectomy; the operation may, in fact, cause an exacerbation of the nephritis. Though there is a difference of opinion, I advise continuous prophylactic penicillin to prevent further streptococcal infections until the urine is normal (*i.e.* until there is no albumin, no excess of red cells in a centrifuged specimen) and the ESR is normal. There should be no limitation of protein in the diet, whether there is residual albuminuria or not.

References

ÅKERRÉN & LINDGREN M. (1955) Investigation concerning early rising in acute haemorrhagic nephritis. *Acta Paediat. Scand.* **151**, 419 and **154**, 245.

JOSEPH M.C. & POLANI P.E. (1958) The effect of rest on acute haemorrhagic nephritis in children. *Guy's Hosp. Rep.* **107**, 500.

McCRORY W.W., FLEISHER D. & SOHN W.B. (1958) The course of acute nephritis in children allowed early resumption of normal physical activity. *Am. J. Dis. Child.* **96**, 576.

NEPHROTIC SYNDROME

A child with the nephrotic syndrome will be under the care of a paediatrician. He may be given corticosteroids or cyclophosphamide.

After loss of oedema, a maintenance dose of prednisolone on three consecutive days a week or at similar intervals may be prescribed until the urine remains albumin-free.

There is no need to keep the child in bed, or to give him a special diet, or to restrict salt in the diet.

It is not normally the practice to give continuous penicillin prophylaxis to prevent infections when the child is receiving corticosteroid treatment, but some advise it. Penicillin is usually given when the initial course of prednisolone in full dosage is being administered.

NEUROBLASTOMA

The child with neuroblastoma will be under the care of a paediatrician. The surgeon may operate to remove the tumour and advise radiotherapy. The paediatrician is likely to prescribe antimitotic drugs such as vincristine and cyclophosphamide. Vitamin B12 used to be given, but it is now known to be useless.

Signs that the condition is deteriorating include increasing pallor, lassitude, purpura, deposits in the orbit, headache, vomiting, cough and abdominal pain.

As in the case of other forms of malignant disease, the family doctor has to try to support the family, especially when the news of the diagnosis is broken to them, and to help the child to live as normal a life as possible.

For *Death and Dying*, see p. 138.

NIGHTMARES

It is normal for children to have an occasional nightmare. Some commonly have a nightmare when starting with an infection, when half awakened by a loud noise, or when they go to bed after a large meal. Repeated and frequent nightmares, *e.g.* one or more every night, are usually associated with insecurity. The family doctor should look for this,

H

in the form of excessive strictness, unkindness, constant nagging or other mismanagement. Medicines will not help.

NOSE – CONGESTION

See also *Allergic Rhinitis, Hay Fever*.

If there is a possibility that the obstruction of the nose is due to deviation of the septum or to polypi, the child should be seen by a specialist.

If the family doctor is satisfied that there is nothing more than nasal congestion, it is better not to prescribe nose drops or other treatment. It is certain that no treatment is required for the nasal congestion of an ordinary cold. It is said that even ½ per cent ephedrine in normal saline drops damages the nasal cilia. Nasal sprays and douches may damage the nasal mucosa and sensitize it to the drugs used. Prolonged use may cause rhinitis. Although some nasal drops momentarily relieve the congestion, they may have a secondary congestant action, so that the child is worse than he would have been if he had used no drops. It is unnecessary to put nose drops into the nose of a young baby. It is better to clean the nose out with pledgets of wet cotton wool. It is highly dangerous to use oily drops, because they may get into the bronchi and cause lipoid pneumonia.

Nose drops should not be used for infants and young children.

References

Anon. (1965) Vasoconstriction solutions for nasal obstruction. *Drug and Therapeutics Bulletin*, 3, 7.

Blue J.A. (1968) Overtreatment of the nasal mucosa. *Ann. Allergy*, 26, 425.

Shaw H. (1964) Nasal drops and sprays. *Prescribers' Journal*, 4, 6.

NOSE, FOREIGN BODY IN

It is often by no means easy for the family doctor to remove the foreign body, and it is easy to push a round object further up the nose when trying to extract the object with no one to restrain the child adequately. If the doctor has any difficulty, he should send the child to hospital for treatment.

OBESITY

It is wrong to ignore excessive weight in a baby or older child, and wrong to tell the mother that 'it is just puppy fat', or 'he will grow out of it'. There is now evidence that excessive weight gain even in the early weeks is apt to be followed by obesity in later years. Eid (1970), working at Sheffield, showed that there is a significant correlation between excessive weight gain as early as 6 weeks of age and obesity in school years. Obesity at school age and beyond is bad physically and emotionally. *It is far better to prevent obesity than to treat it. It is far better to treat it early than to wait until it is fully developed before doing anything about it, for the treatment of obesity is unsatisfactory.* There is evidence that the number of fat cells in the body is determined in the first weeks of life, and that, once determined, the number remains constant; hence excessive weight gain in the early weeks should be avoided.

It may well be that excessive weight gain in the early weeks (*e.g.* in the first two months or so) is due to making bottle feeds too concentrated and to the premature and excessive use of cereals and other carbohydrates (Taitz 1971). The practice of adding rusks and similar carbohydrates to the feeding bottle has nothing to recommend it and should be condemned. The puréed foods purchased in tins all have added cereal, and they contribute to the problem. Later on excessive weight gain may be due to giving too much milk, at the cost of other foodstuffs. Mothers are apt to entertain the totally erroneous idea that the bigger a baby is, the better he is; they are apt to term their horribly fat and therefore ugly babies 'bonny', and think that overweight is desirable. The family doctor can do much to prevent this. Later on, perhaps the most potent cause of obesity is the sweet-eating habit. This should never be started. It is bad for the weight, bad for the teeth, and a waste of money which could more profitably be spent on more useful things. In the same way the habit of eating potato crisps, lollipops and ice-creams at intervals throughout the day should be avoided.

The child's weight should be recorded from birth onwards – perhaps weekly in the first three months, monthly for the remainder of the first year, and then 3-monthly. Any departure from the line on the percentile chart in the way of excessive gain should be dealt with promptly.

In the older child psychological factors are of importance in the causation of obesity. Any form of insecurity may result in overeating. Some children and adults respond to anxiety and tenseness by overeating.

Overeating may be due in part to sibling rivalry; when one child demands more food, the other demands the same, partly so that the sibling cannot have it, and partly because he does not want to be outdone by him. This should be avoided. Overeating, especially in only children, may be related to boredom and loneliness. A mother may encourage overeating or give rich food such as cream in large quantities because she regards the child as delicate.

There are obvious genetic factors. Most fat children have a fat parent – but this may be due more to a familial liking for good food.

Obesity is commonly accompanied by psychological disturbance, because the fat child is teased and given unpleasant nicknames and partly because his mother or father makes remarks to others in his presence about his overweight. I have seen two adolescents who developed anorexia nervosa because of this teasing, and a fat boy who attempted to strangle a girl because she made a practice of sticking pins into him when teasing him for his obesity. It is futile to prescribe a diet for obesity without dealing with the psychological aspects.

As soon as a baby begins to gain weight excessively, the doctor should ensure that the feed is being made up correctly, with no excess of milk powder; sugar should be omitted from the feed unless there is constipation; no cereals should be added to the feeds; no excess total volume of milk should be given – certainly no more than 1½–2 pints (840–1,120 ml.) a day; and puréed fruit, puréed vegetables and puréed meat should be given. It would be better for the mother to prepare the puréed foods herself, if she can, with no sugar or carbohydrate added. Custard, gravy, or banana mashed with milk, may be added to his diet. It is difficult to keep down the carbohydrate content, but every effort should be made to slow down the weight gain.

After infancy I always discuss the diet in the child's presence, telling the overweight mother and father that they also must eat less. I tell the parents that they must see that the child eats less, and the child that he must watch his parents to see that they do the same. It would be most unfair to stop the fat child eating sweets, while his fat mother is eating them throughout the day.

It is impossible to remove fat without removing protein, and protein is needed for growth. In fact, starvation leads to loss of water and protein long before the removal of fat. Overenthusiastic dieting may lead to fatigue and interfere with growth. It is my aim to keep the child's weight static while he grows, rather than reduce his weight. I do not recommend a rigid diet because I know that no child will adhere to it. I prefer to advise the child to stop eating all sweets and chocolates, potato crisps, lollipops and ice-creams, to cut out fruit drinks and sugar in tea or coffee, and to halve the amount of bread and potatoes which he eats. He should also restrict the milk intake to 1 pint per day. He can eat as much fruit and greens as he wishes. Fried foods should be cut down. If he finds it difficult to take the advice because he is hungry, I would prescribe fenfluramine (1 tablet per day at age 6–10, 2 tablets above 10 years). Other appetite suppressants should not be prescribed because of their addictive properties. It is wrong to introduce children to amphetamine or phenmetrazine (Preludin) for this reason.

It is important that the child should increase the amount of exercise taken. The older child may be encouraged to join the 'Weight-Watchers'.

Follow-up is essential, with constant reminders about the need to adhere to the diet, for relapse is not only common, it is usual.

Fenfluramine (Ponderax) is supplied in 20 mg. tablets and should be given in the following doses:
6–8 years: 1 tablet daily.
8–12 years: 1 tablet b.d.

References

Eid E.E. (1970) A follow up study of physical growth of children who had excessive weight gain in the first six months of life with special reference to its relation to obesity. *Brit. Med. J.* **2**, 74.

Taitz L.S. (1971) Infantile overnutrition among artificially fed infants in the Sheffield region. *Brit. Med. J.* **1**, 315.

OTITIS EXTERNA

If the otitis externa is due to a purulent discharge from the ear, the underlying otitis media should be treated in the usual way with antibiotics, and the discharge should be removed by wisps of cotton wool. Cotton wool plugs should be avoided because free drainage is required. Hydrogen peroxide drops may be used to help to remove debris, aided by pledgets of cotton wool.

If there is no associated otitis media, the otitis externa may be treated by hydrocortisone and neomycin ear drops, BNF, discontinuing these as soon as possible because of the risk of sensitization. Alternative treatments include aluminium acetate ear drops (NF) or corticosteroid ointment. Locorten-Vioform ear drops (quinoline and corticosteroid) are favoured by some because they carry less risk of sensitization. For candida infection one would use nystatin drops.

If the infection is deep, it would be wise to give phenoxymethyl penicillin by mouth 125–250 mg. q.d. for a week.

Pain may be relieved by aspirin.

Syringing should not be allowed until the otitis externa has cleared.

OTITIS MEDIA

Immediately otitis media is diagnosed, antibiotic treatment should be instituted. Despite the finding that some cases are due to Haemophilus Influenzae, penicillin G seems to be satisfactory in the great majority of cases. It is usually advisable to begin with an injection (*e.g.* of Triplopen), in order to ensure rapid action, and to follow this two days later by phenoxymethyl penicillin by mouth (125–250 mg. 6-hourly by mouth, day and night) for eight days (*i.e.* for the equivalent of ten days, when the injection is included). It is essential that the penicillin should not be discontinued sooner, for relapse is apt to occur if treatment lasts less than ten days. Because of the possibility of a Haemophilus Influenzae infection, some prefer ampicillin. *It is futile to prescribe ear drops, with the sole possible exception of analgesic ear drops if there is much pain* (e.g. *auralgicin, which consists of benzocaine, ephedrine, phenazone, chlorbutol, glycerine and potassium hydroxyquinoline), but I have never found it necessary to prescribe them myself. The possibility that these drops may sensitize the skin must be remembered. It is totally inadequate to treat acute otitis media by ear drops alone. Yet vast numbers of prescriptions are written every year for ear drops for otitis media, at enormous expense to the country.* In 1968, 1,303,700 prescriptions were written in England and Wales for only three preparations of ear drops – enough to provide 30 drops for every pre-school child in the country.

If a drum is found to be bulging, the child should be seen immediately by an ear, nose and throat surgeon for myringotomy. With prompt treatment, bulging and certainly rupture should not occur.

If the drum has ruptured, and there is a purulent discharge, it is wrong to insert a cotton wool plug in the ear. It is far better to allow the discharge to drain. An antibiotic, such as ampicillin, is essential.

If there is recurrent otitis media, the possibility of adenoids should be considered. If there is mouthbreathing, postnasal obstruction, nasal speech and a postnasal discharge causing cough at night, the child should be referred to an ear, nose and throat surgeon for an opinion.

A common and serious mistake in the management of acute otitis media is to see the child once and not to see him again to make sure that the treatment has been effective.

OVERACTIVITY

Excessive overactivity is due to a variety of causes, including prenatal or natal anoxia, mental subnormality or excessive restriction. More often than not, the child merely takes after one of his parents who in childhood behaved in the same way. Most if not all overactive children lose their overactivity as they mature.

Drug treatment is rarely necessary, but if one does have to prescribe something, because the overactivity is really excessive and intolerable, the most useful drug is dextroamphetamine, beginning with 0·1 mg./kg. in one dose only, in the morning, increasing as necessary to 0·25 mg./kg. Dextroamphetamine frequently has a paradoxical effect in overactive children, and successfully quietens them. It should certainly not be used for an older child, because of the risk of addiction. In fact, it would be unnecessary, because the overactivity nearly always disappears as the child gets older. Other drugs worth trying are methylphenidate (Ritalin), 0·2 mg./kg. in a single morning dose, increasing if necessary to 0·5 mg./kg., or chlordiazepoxide (Librium) 0·25–1·0 mg./kg. An alternative is thioridazine (Melleril) 20–60 mg. per day. Meprobamate is not useful for the purpose. Phenobarbitone should be avoided, because it may have the paradoxical effect of making the child worse.

References

MILLICHAP G. (1968) Overactivity. *J. Am. Med. Ass.* 206, 1527.
WERRY J.S. (1968) Developmental hyperactivity. *Pediatric Clinics N. America,* 15, 581.

PAIN

See also *Headache, Abdominal Pain.*

The treatment must depend on the cause.

Paracetamol may be used if the child is allergic to aspirin. It has the advantage that it is less likely to cause peptic ulceration than aspirin, but it is more expensive. It has no antirheumatic activity.

I suggest the drug paracetamol BPC be prescribed rather than the same drug, which is usually more expensive, under proprietary names.

Paracetamol is made up in 500 mg. tablets; between the ages of 6–12 years the dose is 250–500 mg.

Paracetamol has the following trade names: Panadol, Tabalgin, Calpol, Cetal, Eneril, Febrilix.

PANCREAS, FIBROCYSTIC DISEASE OF THE

It is essential that the suspected diagnosis of fibrocystic disease of the pancreas should be confirmed by special investigations (*e.g.* a sweat test) in the hospital, in order that the correct treatment can be given. The child will remain under the supervision of the specialist.

The treatment may be discussed under the following headings:

(1) Nutrition

Every effort must be made to achieve good nutritional status. A high-calorie high-protein diet should be given, with additional Vitamins A and D (*e.g.* as Abidec). Some now advocate a diet containing medium chain triglycerides (Trufood) or Alembicol D in order to decrease the steatorrhoea.

Pancreatin is given in order to promote absorption of protein. The dose is regulated by the state of the stools; if looseness remains, the dose should be increased.

(2) Antibiotics

There is a difference of opinion as to whether continuous antibiotic therapy should be given to all children in order to prevent infection, or whether antibiotics should only be given for the treatment of acute or chronic chest infection. I prefer the latter course, unless chest infection is already established, because continuous antibiotic therapy is apt to result in the overgrowth of other organisms. If the specialist is able to recover the predominant organism in the chest, the treatment can be adjusted accordingly. For any acute infection, intensive antibiotic treatment should be given for two or three weeks. The antibiotic most likely to be used for prolonged prophylaxis would be ampicillin. Tetracyclines would be avoided because of the effect on the teeth.

Antibiotic aerosols are recommended by some. The antibiotics used include neomycin, penicillin, colistin, kanamycin and gentamycin. Some of these are expensive. The danger is the development of allergy.

(3) Maintenance of the airway

Breathing exercises and postural drainage may help (p. 105).

Potassium iodide may help to liquefy thick secretions, but prolonged usage may cause goitre formation. It is probably better avoided.

A mist tent may help at night, using acetyl cysteine (Airbron) 2–5 ml. of a 20 per cent solution two to five times a day, or propylene glycol 10 per cent, glycerol 3 per cent with water 87 per cent. Some advocate acetyl cysteine aerosol (2–5 ml. of a 20 per cent solution two to five times a day); this may have a slight bronchoconstrictor action, and should not be given for a wheezing child. The value of the mist tent with acetyl cysteine is doubtful.

Bronchial spasm may be relieved by bronchodilator drugs such as theophylline.

(4) Treatment of complications

A rectal prolapse is treated by replacing the prolapsed bowel in the knee chest position, and then strapping the buttocks together. (See also *Rectal Prolapse*, p. 229.)

Faecal impaction is treated by an enema, followed by liquid paraffin.

Antrum infection, which is common, sometimes with polyp formation and deafness, is treated by the ear, nose and throat specialist.

In hot weather, salt loss is treated by giving additional 2–4 g. of sodium chloride per day.

(5) Treatment of the whole child

If at all possible, the child should attend an ordinary school rather than a special one. Overprotection should be avoided. A child with severe fibrocystic disease of the pancreas is apt to be spoilt and the subject of favouritism, so that he is given all his own way without discipline. He should be immunized against the usual infections, in particular pertussis and measles.

It is useful for the parents to join the parents' association. Parents may receive useful help from The Cystic Fibrosis Research Foundation Trust, Stuart House, 1 Tudor Street, London EC4.

Preparations

Pancreatin preparations differ considerably in price, and the more expensive ones (*e.g.* Cotazym) offer no convincing advantages over the National Formulary and BP preparations.

Pancreatin strong BP (Pancrex V) is a satisfactory preparation; the doses are as follows:

Pancrex V powder

Up to 1 year   0·5–1·0 g. with meals.

1–12 years   2·0 g. with meals.

Puberty   4·0 g. with meals.

Capsules (340 mg.): contents of capsule emptied onto food or mixed with food.

Up to 1 year   1–3 capsules.

1–12 years   3–6 capsules.

Pancrex V forte (200 mg. tablets = 1 g. pancreatin BP)

6–12 years   3–6 tablets with meals.

Acetyl cysteine (Airbron) is for use in an atomizer connected to a pressure air-line. It is not suitable for hand nebulizers. It should be given in doses of 2–5 ml. 3–4 times per day.

When ampoules are opened they must be stored in a refrigerator and used within hours.

References

ANON. (1968) Pancreatin. *Drug and Therapeutics Bulletin*, 6, 82.

ANON. (1969) Medium chain triglycerides. *Drug and Therapeutics Bulletin*, 7, 43.

GREENBERGER N.J. & SKILLMAN T. (1969) Medium chain triglycerides. *New Engl. J. Med.* 280, 1045.

PARAPHIMOSIS

A paraphimosis can be reduced by applying the first finger of each hand behind the swollen ring of the prepuce and the thumb to the oiled glans; the glans is pushed back and the foreskin is pulled over it. If necessary, the foreskin is first wrapped in gauze wrung out of iced water in order to reduce the congestion. If this fails, hyaluronidase (1,500 International Units) is dissolved in 4 ml. of 1 per cent xylocaine and injected 'round the clock' into the oedematous ring. The penis is wrapped in gauze wrung out of iced water. The swelling subsides in a few minutes.

PECTUS EXCAVATUM

See *Funnel Chest*.

PEDICULOSIS

An emulsion containing benzyl benzoate 12·5 per cent, benzocaine 2 per cent and dicophane (DDT) 1 per cent is rubbed into the scalp, making sure that all hair is wet with it; the eyes are covered up during the treatment. The scalp is left unwashed for 24 hours. Combs and brushes are thoroughly washed, along with the pillows and bedding.

Alternatively, 2 per cent gamma benzene hexachloride BPC (Lorexane lotion or shampoo). 15 ml. are applied to the scalp with a minimum of friction, leaving the hair unwashed for 24 hours. There is no need to comb the nits out. A further treatment is given ten days later.

Other members of the family with nits should be treated.

PHENYLKETONURIA

The diagnosis and treatment of phenylketonuria is highly specialized and requires expert laboratory investigation. An affected child requires constant supervision by a paediatrician.

The family doctor should know that if the serum phenylalanine is allowed to drop too low, the child is apt to lose his appetite, to become lethargic and to lose weight; he may become lethargic, anaemic, and develop hypoglycaemia and a rash.

If the serum phenylalanine is allowed to rise too high, the child is apt to become irritable and to cry excessively (if he is a baby). A febrile illness commonly results in a rise of the serum phenylalanine.

Failure to give adequate vitamin cover, in the way of ketovite tablets and syrup, results in an erythematous rash in the perineal region, on the face and scalp.

It is unknown whether the special diet can be discontinued, and if so at what age this can be done. It may be that by the age of 6 or 7 the child can take ordinary food without harm. The paediatrician may make the experiment of introducing ordinary food and carefully observing the child in order to determine whether harm is being done.

PICA

Pica or dirt-eating may occur in imitation of others, including the parents, or as an attention-seeking device if the parents show great anxiety about it. For instance, I have had patients who ate live snails or roundworms, who filled the mouth with stones, or who drank drain water, all as attention-seeking devices. Though it is common in normal children, especially amongst the poor, it is particularly common in mentally subnormal ones. A mentally normal child characteristically takes everything to the mouth from about 5 to 12 months of age, and thereafter ceases this practice, but a mentally subnormal child does it much longer.

The treatment must depend on the cause, dealing with insecurity, if any, and trying to stop the parents displaying anxiety at the child's antics.

It is as well to determine (by laboratory means, normally the blood lead estimation) whether a child with pica has acquired lead poisoning.

PIGEON CHEST

No treatment is required.

PNEUMONIA

The infecting organism may be a penicillin-resistant staphylococcus, and full laboratory help may be needed. The infant may require oxygen, hydration and digoxin, so that hospital treatment is required. The older child with lobar pneumonia can often be nursed satisfactorily at home. The treatment of choice is penicillin (*e.g.* triplopen) once a day for two days, followed by oral phenoxymethyl penicillin 125–250 mg. 6-hourly according to age for eight days. It is important that after treatment an X-ray of the chest should be taken, in order to ensure that resolution is complete.

There is no need to give a cough medicine. Chest pain due to pleurisy is rarely a problem in a child. It is not usually necessary to prescribe anything to promote sleep, but Chloral would be safe for the purpose.

Recurrent pneumonia suggests the possibility of chronic antrum infection, fibrocystic disease of the pancreas, bronchiectasis or asthma, and investigation for these is indicated.

POISONING ACCIDENTS

Most cases of poisoning should be sent to hospital immediately. The doctor must never be misled by the apparently good condition of the child, for the child may be in the dangerous latent period (*e.g.* after ferrous sulphate, salicylate or diphenoxylate [lomotil] poisoning). The child should be transported to hospital in the 'spanking' position – in the prone, so that if he vomits, inhalation of vomit is unlikely. If necessary, the child's mouth should be sucked out by a mucus catheter.

The family doctor may think that it is desirable to induce vomiting. *Vomiting must never be induced after kerosene (paraffin) poisoning or after the ingestion of white spirit or other petroleum products.* For other conditions vomiting may be induced, only when the child is in the prone position and conscious, by the insertion of the blunt handle of a spoon into the throat, or by administering a salt solution (two tablespoonsful of salt in a tumblerful of water). Some have advocated the administration of 15–20 ml. (an average tablespoonful) of syrup ipecacuanha, but others think that this is unwise. This should not be given to a child who has ingested a corrosive substance or a petroleum derivative. No attempt should be made to wash his stomach out in the home.

If the child is shocked, his lower limbs are raised. He must not be overheated if he has a subnormal temperature; hot-water bottles should not be used.

If the child is having a convulsion, paraldehyde 1 ml. per year up to 5 ml. are given intramuscularly into the thigh. If the convulsions are due to imipramine or amitriptyline, intramuscular phenobarbitone may be given. The poisonous substance taken by the child should be sent with him to the hospital.

Below are some further suggestions.

For respiratory depression, one should ensure that there is an airway, apply mouth-to-mouth resuscitation if necessary, and transfer him to the hospital in the spank position.

For barbiturate poisoning, analeptic drugs are not advised.

For fungus poisoning, induce vomiting.

For ingested bleaching agents – empty the stomach and leave milk in.

For detergents – leave milk in.

A stomach tube should not be passed if a caustic substance has been taken, because of the risk of perforation.

For carbon monoxide poisoning, provide fresh air, artificial respiration if necessary, and if possible oxygen. If there is a near-by centre where hyperbaric oxygen can be given, he should be transported there immediately.

For caustic substances on the skin, remove the contaminated clothes and wash with soap and water; but if the caustic material is pure carbolic, water should not be used.

For a caustic substance in the eye, hold the child with the face upright under the cold water tap and irrigate the eye.

When the family doctor urgently needs advice while waiting for an ambulance to take a child to hospital, or when he wants to know whether a particular substance is poisonous or not, he can obtain the information by asking for the Poisons Information Service at the following centres:

	Code	Telephone
Belfast	[0232–]	40503
Cardiff	[0222–]	33101
Edinburgh	[031–]	229 2477
Leeds	[0532–]	32799
London	[01–]	407 7600
Manchester	[061–]	740 2254
Newcastle	[0632–]	25131

Reference

MATTHEW H. & LAWSON A.A.H. (1970) *Treatment of Common Acute Poisoning*. Edinburgh, Livingstone.

POLIOMYELITIS

A child with meningism would be sent to hospital immediately, in order to eliminate pyogenic meningitis; and a child with suspected poliomyelitis would be sent to hospital. When a decision is being made, strict bed rest is desirable, for Horstmann showed that in the prodromal stage of poliomyelitis, the amount of exercise did not affect the eventual outcome, but that physical exertion in the forty-eight hours after the onset of meningism increased the risk of paralysis. Ritchie Russell made the same observation at Oxford.

It is hoped that the family doctor will do his best to ensure that all the children in his practice are immunized against poliomyelitis.

The period of infectivity is from 3 weeks before the development of symptoms until 2 weeks after their development, provided that the temperature is normal.

Incubation period: 4–30 days (especially 7–14 days).

Quarantine is probably not required; some may demand it.

References

HORSTMANN D.M. (1950) Physical activity and paralysis in poliomyelitis. *J. Am. Med. Ass.* **142**, 236.

RUSSELL W.R. (1947) Poliomyelitis. *Brit. Med. J.* **2**, 1023.

PREAURICULAR SINUS

Surgeons advise treatment of a preauricular sinus at the age of 2 or 3 years on the grounds that if it is left alone, infection and boil formation is apt to occur.

PREMATURITY (Low birth-weight babies)

Small babies (*e.g.* below 4 lb. in weight) should normally be looked after in hospital because of the feeding problems which they present. A baby who is small for dates may be more mature than a premature baby of the same birth weight, and easier to manage at home.

Low birth-weight babies, epecially those born before term, are thermolabile; they are more liable than others to be chilled and to suffer cold injury, and more liable than others to be overheated. Hence a room with a carefully regulated temperature is needed, around 70–75° F, and the baby's temperature must be recorded two or three times a day, maintaining it at 97–98°. There is no need for extra humidity.

As for the feeding of the low birth-weight baby, there is no evidence that any one artificial feed is better than another, except that it is wise to start with a half-cream milk. We have found half-cream National Dried Milk or half-cream Cow and Gate or Ostermilk No. 1 entirely satisfactory; I do not wish to imply that other dried milks or evaporated milk are not also satisfactory.

The low birth weight must not be underfed. He needs relatively more per lb. of body weight than a full-term baby.

The following are the usual quantities of properly reconstituted feeds which he will require:

Day	2	4	6	8	10	14	21	28
Oz. per lb. per day	$\frac{1}{2}$	1	$1\frac{1}{2}$	2	$2\frac{1}{2}$	3	$3\frac{1}{2}$	4
Approximate (ml.) per kilo	30	60	90	120	150	180	210	240

I recommend that the premature baby be given his first feed of boiled water within twelve hours or so of birth, followed at the next feed by milk, a few drops, increasing at each feed. There is no rule as to the frequency of his feeds. It would be sensible to feed him 3-hourly by day and perhaps 4-hourly by night in the early days. Self-demand feeding is not feasible, because premature babies cannot be relied upon to demand feeds. When he reaches the weight of an average full-term baby, the method of feeding is adjusted accordingly.

Additional vitamins are added when he is 6 weeks of age or so (*e.g.* Abidec drops 5 twice a day) and ferrous sulphate (*e.g.* 60 mg. per day) to prevent anaemia. These are continued throughout the first year.

225

PRICKLY HEAT

This annoying skin condition may result merely from overclothing; I have seen it in a cold spell in midwinter. If the child is overclothed, the mother should be given the necessary advice. If the weather is hot, tepid sponging several times a day, followed by the application of calamine lotion and then talcum powder, would be suitable. It is better to avoid ointment. A lotion containing tannic acid 2 per cent with alcohol 20 per cent in aq. dest. is useful.

PRURITUS

The common causes of general itching are scabies, eczema, urticaria, and lichen planus. Pruritus ani or vulvae may result from candida infection, which normally responds to nystatin cream.

Pruritus may be aggravated by overtreatment. For instance, an antihistamine cream is likely to sensitize the skin and increase the itching. Benzocaine ointment applied to a fissure in ano may sensitize the skin with the same result; lignocaine ointment is to be preferred, being less likely to sensitize. Even corticosteroid ointment may occasionally prolong itching around the vulva or anus. Itching around the vulva may be due to degreasing by constant washing with soap and water. Pruritus ani may be due to threadworms, and if so, the infection should be treated.

If a child has persistent pruritus, and an obvious cause cannot be found and successfully treated, he should be referred to a dermatologist.

PSORIASIS

The child with psoriasis should be referred to a specialist for advice about the treatment. Sneddon (1964) advised that the child's limbs should be soaked in a warm bath, the scales scrubbed off with a soft nailbrush, and ammoniated mercury ointment with tar applied on tube gauze (solution of coal tar 10 parts, ammoniated mercury 2·25 parts, yellow soft paraffin to 100 parts), or 1 per cent tar in zinc ointment BP applied morning and night, or dithranol ¼ per cent in Lassar's paste BPC. This should not be applied to the face or flexures. For the scalp he recommended washing the hair with 1–2 per cent cetrimide every night, followed by the application of 2–4 per cent liquor picis carb in Boots E.45. If there are hard scales on the scalp, an ointment of 3 per cent sulphur and 3 per cent salicylic acid in soft paraffin rubbed in at night for one or two nights is effective. For the face he recommended betamethazone valeriate ointment (Betnovate). For hard scales, Calnurid may be effective.

References

ANON. (1971) Calnurid, a urea cream for the skin. *Drug and Therapeutics Bulletin*, 9, 29.
SNEDDON I.B. (1968) Treatment of psoriasis. *Prescribers' Journal*, 8, 58.
SNEDDON, I.B. & CHURCH R.E. (1964) *Practical Dermatology*. London, Arnold.

PUBERTY

Delayed puberty may be a mere normal variation, following a familial pattern, and no treatment is required. If there is doubt about this, the child should be referred to a paediatrician for diagnosis.

Excessively early puberty may be due to a variety of causes, and expert help should always be sought. In the case of the girl, the most likely cause is constitutional precocious puberty, a normal variation, but special investigations are needed to confirm this diagnosis. In the boy the cause is usually much more serious, in the form of a tumour of the hypothalamus, adrenal or testis.

PURPURA

The diagnosis must be established by the hospital in order that appropriate treatment can be given.

If the child has anaphylactoid (Henoch-Schönlein) purpura, there is no specific treatment. Corticosteroids are not of value except *possibly* for the relief of abdominal pain.

If the child has idiopathic thrombocytopenic purpura, the specialist is likely to prescribe corticosteroids, and if they fail, azathiaprine. If the platelet count fails to rise after about two years, splenectomy will be considered. Paediatricians are reluctant to advise splenectomy in the first five years of life, because after removal of the spleen young children are more likely to develop septicaemia or other serious infections. It is customary to prescribe continuous prophylactic penicillin up to school age if it has become necessary to remove the spleen from young children.

PYELONEPHRITIS

See *Urinary Tract Infection* (p. 268).

PYLORIC STENOSIS, CONGENITAL

The treatment for congenital pyloric stenosis is the Ramstedt operation. This effects a rapid cure and the child is normally discharged home on about the third postoperative day. It is wrong to attempt medical treatment with atropine methylnitrate (Eumydrin); it is true that if the child survives, the vomiting will eventually cease, but until then there is a constant danger that he will inhale vomit and die as a result. It is far better to cure the child immediately by surgery. The operation has virtually no mortality.

As a diagnosis of pylorospasm is probably invariably wrong, it would be a mistake to treat vomiting as pylorospasm.

QUARRELSOMENESS AND AGGRESSIVENESS

A mother may be worried because her child frequently quarrels with his siblings or with a neighbour's children. It is important that she should know that quarrelsomeness and aggressiveness are normal features of the developing child. She should resist the temptation of always stepping into the fray and trying to settle disputes, though she may step in when she sees that the limit of tolerance is being reached and a fight is imminent. The child is learning something which the only child misses – that he cannot have all his own way; he has to learn to give and take. It is much better for him that he should learn that at home than that he should learn it much more painfully after he has started school.

Excessive aggressiveness can be a troublesome behaviour problem. It may be in part an attention-seeking device, the child having discovered that his behaviour is attracting a great deal of attention and is causing much fuss and anxiety. When a mother says, 'I have tried everything to stop it', she needs to know that that is the reason for the child's bad behaviour; she should ignore it as far as possible, stepping in only if he seems to be about to hurt someone but otherwise showing no interest in his behaviour. In addition, she must try to make him feel more secure and important. Punishment will achieve nothing but harm.

Some of his aggressiveness may be an inherited trait. Some may be the result of imitating a sibling. Some may be due to boredom, fatigue or even hunger. If the family doctor is asked for advice about a child's aggressiveness, the whole management will have to be reviewed. Medicine will not help.

RECTAL PROLAPSE

The cause of rectal prolapse is usually unknown. It may occur in association with meningomyelocele or extrophy of the bladder, in both cases as a result of a lax anal sphincter. It may be associated with fibrocystic disease of the pancreas or severe malnutrition. In most cases, however, there is no evidence of underlying disease.

The majority undergo spontaneous remission if the stools are kept soft but not liquid, so that straining is avoided. In cases not responding to such conservative treatment, the paediatric surgeon may inject 30 per cent saline into the wall of the rectum. Kay & Zachary (1970) described 51 cases successfully treated by this method – 40 by a single injection, 8 by two injections and the remaining 3 by three injections.

Reference

KAY N.R.M. & ZACHARY R.B. (1970) The treatment of rectal prolapse in children with injections of 30 per cent saline solutions. *J. Pediat. Surgery,* **5,** 334.

RHEUMATIC FEVER

In my opinion a child with rheumatic fever should always be treated in hospital. Not all will agree, because there is disagreement about the best treatment.

The first problem concerns the optimum dosage of salicylates. On the basis of research done in Sheffield and elsewhere, I recommend large dosage to maintain a serum salicylate level of around 30 mg. per cent. This is a potentially dangerous treatment which requires constant laboratory help in the way of repeated serum salicylate levels, and constant supervision in order that early signs of salicylate intoxication, in the form of over-ventilation, may be detected. It would be wrong to give salicylates in high dosage at home because of the considerable danger of salicylate intoxication and death. We showed, as have others, that for the best results a high serum salicylate level is needed.

The second problem concerns corticosteroid treatment. Whereas probably no paediatrician would wish to withhold salicylates, albeit in low dosage, many would withhold corticosteroids except only for severe cases. Research in Sheffield and elsewhere indicated that corticosteroids are of great value, especially in combination with salicylates in high dosage, in reducing the duration of rheumatic activity. The combined treatment led to a far more rapid fall of the ESR to normal than corti-costeroids alone, and still more than salicylates alone.

The following were our findings in a random sample study of 141 children.

The mean duration of an elevated ESR

	Days
Untreated	116
Salicylates in low dosage	58
Salicylates in high dosage	51
Corticosteroids alone	25·8
Corticosteroids and salicylates in low dosage	18·5
Corticosteroids and salicylates in high dosage	16·2

By the end of the second and sixth week, the following were the percentages with a normal ESR.

	Normal ESR (percentage)	
	second week	*sixth week*
No treatment	0	29·6
Salicylates in low dosage	6·7	60·0
Salicylates in high dosage	14·2	79·0
Corticosteroids alone	47·8	91·5
Corticosteroids and salicylates in low dosage	50·0	100·0
Corticosteroids and salicylates in high dosage	81·8	100·0

Unfortunately a joint Anglo-American study did not confirm that corticosteroids alone were of value. Nevertheless, I think that it is true to say that the majority of paediatricians who have written about the subject advocate the use of corticosteroids for severe cases. It would seem logical to me to argue that if corticosteroids are important for the severe case, they should also be used for the milder one.

It is important, if possible, to prevent cardiac damage. We have never seen a child in whom a cardiac murmur developed during corticosteroid treatment, but we have seen eight or more children in whom a murmur developed while on salicylates alone. It would also seem desirable to stop rheumatic activity as soon as possible; and our figures showed that the combined treatments achieved that.

A third problem concerns the duration of bed rest required. In recent years it has become recognized that prolonged rest in bed is quite unnecessary and, in fact, may do more harm than good. Grossman (1968) divided 122 children with acute rheumatic fever into two groups, both treated by prednisolone. One group was kept in bed for 15 weeks, and the other until the ESR was normal (usually 2–3 weeks); there was no difference in the outcome. There have been several publications describing similar findings. Gibson & Fisher (1958) allowed 44 children with active rheumatic carditis full activity in the ward as soon as they were well enough (usually within 48 hours), and there were no ill results. May Wilson (1962), who has extensive experience of the treatment of rheumatic fever in children, allows her patients to be up and about within two or three weeks of instituting corticosteroid treatment. Browse (1965) wrote that one thing that lying down does not do is to rest the heart; it increases the cardiac output and the work done by the heart. He wrote: 'The main reason for the use of rest in the treatment of rheumatic fever appears to stem from a fear that it may be unethical to treat it in any other way.' It has long been our practice in Sheffield to allow the child to get up to go to the lavatory from the day of admission, and to allow him out of bed otherwise as soon as the ESR falls to normal. Robertson *et al.* (1946) wrote: 'Based on our observations of more than 200 cases of rheumatic fever, it is our opinion that greater rest was obtained by permitting more freedom for activity, such as sitting in or out of bed and walking to the latrine.'

Once all rheumatic activity has ceased, normal exercise is allowed. There should be no restriction with regard to games, even though there is a residual organic cardiac murmur.

Continuous prophylactic penicillin is given for several years, at least into adolescence, in order to prevent recurrence. This can be given in the form of penicillin G (200,000 units twice a day), or phenoxymethyl penicillin 125 mg. twice a day.

References

BROWSE N.L. (1965) *The Physiology and Pathology of Bed Rest.* Springfield, Charles Thomas.

DUMAN L.J., GITHENS J.H. & HOFFMAN M.S. (1957) Role of rest in treatment of rheumatic fever. *J. Am. Med. Ass.* 164, 1435.

GIBSON M.L. & FISHER G.R. (1958) Early ambulation in rheumatic fever. *Am. J. Dis. Child.* 96, 575.

GROSSMAN B.J. (1968) Early ambulation in the treatment of acute rheumatic fever. *Am. J. Dis. Child.* 115, 557.

HOLT K.S., ILLINGWORTH R.S., LORBER J. & RENDLE-SHORT J. (1954) Cortisone and salicylates in rheumatic fever. *Lancet,* 2, 1144.

ILLINGWORTH R.S., BURKE J., DOXIADIS S.A., LORBER J., PHILPOTT M.G. & STONE D.G.H. (1954) Salicylates in rheumatic fever; an attempt to assess their value. *Quart. J. Med.* 23, 177.

ILLINGWORTH R.S., LORBER J., HOLT K.S. & RENDLE-SHORT J. (1957) Acute rheumatic fever in children: A comparison of six forms of treatment of 200 cases. *Lancet,* 2, 653.

LENDRUM B.L., SIMON A.J. & MACK I. (1959) Effect on the child's heart of early resump-
tion of normal physical activity following acute rheumatic fever as evaluated 2 to
14 years later. *Am. J. Dis. Child.* 98, 519.
NASSAU E. & ARON A. (1959) Early ambulation in patients with acute rheumatic fever.
Ann. Paediat. 193, 101.
RHEUMATIC FEVER WORKING PARTY OF THE MEDICAL RESEARCH COUNCIL OF GREAT
BRITAIN (1955) Treatment of acute rheumatic fever in children. *Brit. Med. J.* 1, 555.
ROBERTSON H.F., SCHMIDT R.E. & FEIRING W. (1946) The therapeutic value of early
physical activity in rheumatic fever. *Am. J. Med. Sc.* 211, 67.
WILSON M.G. (1962) *Advances in Rheumatic Fever 1940-1961.* Commonwealth Fund,
Harper, New York.

RHEUMATOID ARTHRITIS

Although the specialist should see the child with suspected rheumatoid
arthritis in order to confirm the diagnosis and advise treatment, it is the
family doctor who has the opportunity of guiding the parents with regard
to the management of the child, and of observing the child's progress so
that if necessary the advised treatment can be reconsidered.

The child with rheumatoid arthritis should not be kept in bed unless
the arthritis of ankle or knee is so painful that the child cannot bear the
weight and walk. If symptoms are so severe, the paediatrician should
reassess the child and consider the administration of a short course of
corticosteroids. Such a case would be exceptional. Normally the child
with rheumatoid arthritis should be up and about, partly because if his
joints are rested they are apt to become stiff, and partly because the child
is happier when ambulant. It has been shown that bed rest does no good
and may do harm. Ansell & Bywaters (1963) wrote from their extensive
experience: 'Every effort should be made to get the patient up walking
every day, even when fever is present, provided his general health is
otherwise reasonable. Only under rare conditions of severe constitutional
manifestations, severe pain, severe hip involvement, or when flexion
deformities of knees and hips are aggravated by ambulation, should the
child be confined to bed, and then only for short periods. We have seen
too much irreversible damage done by bed rest to think that it has an
important part to play in the treatment of Still's disease. Muscles and
bones waste, joints ankylose, contractures, calculi and bed sores develop,
and above all, time is lost.' Calabro (1970) in a valuable review of the
treatment of rheumatoid arthritis in children, wrote: 'It is preferable that

growing young patients have a little discomfort, even pain, than the alternative complications of prolonged inactivity – muscle atrophy, bedsores, skeletal demineralization and renal calculus.'

Physiotherapy is of importance for the prevention of contractures and deformity. All affected joints should be put through a full range of movement several times a day. The physiotherapist will show the parents how this is done. In addition the physiotherapist may advise about ways of getting the child to use affected hands – by finger paints, drawing, plasticine and building toys. The tricycle may help the child to use his ankles and knees.

The eye specialist should examine the eyes not less than 6-monthly with a slit lamp, in order to detect early signs of iridocyclitis, a complication affecting some 10 per cent of all cases, but as many as 30 per cent of children with the monoarthritic form. The condition is symptomless at first. Prompt treatment with corticosteroids is likely to save the child's vision.

Morning stiffness is a feature of rheumatoid arthritis. A warm bath in the morning may help the child to loosen up.

The most useful medicine in aspirin, in a dose of 50 mg./kg./day in four divided doses for a child up to 5 years. Aspirin is preferable to proprietary preparations, which have no special advantages and are more expensive. If a child is receiving both aspirin and corticosteroids, the withdrawal of corticosteroids may precipitate salicylism.

Corticosteroids should be used only if everything else fails, or for the treatment of a severe acute episode or for iridocyclitis. They should be discontinued as soon as possible, *e.g.* after a fortnight's course, partly because of their side effects, including osteoporosis, and partly because the child becomes dependent on them. One would give prednisolone in a dose of 0·1–0·4 mg./kg./day. An intraarticular corticosteroid injection for a troublesome monarthritis may be administered by a specialist.

Chloroquin was recommended for a time, but found to be too dangerous because of the effect on the eye, in causing corneal opacities and sometimes an irreversible retinal change.

Mepacrine is sometimes of value, but it has the disadvantage that it stains the skin yellow. It has to be taken for several weeks.

Butazolidin and allied drugs are not used in children because of their serious effects on the bone marrow.

Indomethacin is little used because of its side effects, and research has shown that it is no more effective than aspirin and yet is considerably more expensive. It is not recommended for children.

Ibufenac has been withdrawn. Flufenamic acid and ibuprofen offered no advantage over aspirin. The same is true of mefenamic acid.

Gold therapy has a place in the treatment of refractory cases, in spite of the many possible side effects. It would be administered by a specialist.

It is important that the child should as far as possible be treated as a a normal child, overprotection and favouritism being avoided. The child should be kept off school only if absolutely necessary. The parents should be reassured that, although nothing can be promised, the majority of affected children 'cure' themselves with no residual disability. Unfortunately in some the deformity of the joint remains.

References

ANON. (1966) Drugs for rheumatoid arthritis. *Drug and Therapeutics Bulletin*, 4, 21.
ANON. (1966) Ibufenac. *Drug and Therapeutics Bulletin*, 4, 46.
ANON. (1967) Flufenamic acid in rheumatoid arthritis. *Drug and Therapeutics Bulletin*, 5, 103.
ANON. (1969) Brufen in rheumatoid arthritis. *Drug and Therapeutics Bulletin*, 7, 35.
ANSELL B. & BYWATERS E.G.L. (1963) Rheumatoid arthritis. *Pediat. Clin. N. America*, 10, 921.
CALABRO J.J. (1970) Management of Juvenile Rheumatoid Arthritis. *J. Pediat.* 77, 355.
PRESCOTT L.E. (1968) Mefenamic acid. *Prescribers' Journal*, 8, 109.

RICKETS

Vitamin D is added to dried milks and cereals by manufacturers, and because of the risk of hypercalcaemia owing to excess of Vitamin D, I prescribe codliver oil only for fully breast-fed babies. Opinions differ as to the optimum prophylactic dose of Vitamin D, but it is probable that it is less than has been commonly thought. About 150 I.Units are probably sufficient, and that quantity is more than adequately covered by the amount added by manufacturers to dried milks and cereals.

The clinical diagnosis of rickets should always be confirmed by radiological and biochemical investigation, and hence every child with suspected rickets should be referred to a paediatrician. In the first place, radiological examination in a child with suspected mild rickets commonly reveals no abnormality at all; secondly, investigation may reveal some other less common condition, such as Blount's disease; and thirdly, even if the diagnosis of rickets is confirmed, laboratory investigation is necessary to determine whether the child has nutritional rickets or rickets due to other metabolic conditions such as an abnormal aminoaciduria.

The treatment of nutritional rickets consists of Vitamin D in a dose of 300–500 units per day for a month. If the home is a poor one, as it is likely to be if the child has been allowed to develop nutritional rickets, one cannot rely on the Vitamin D being given. There is then much to be said for a single intramuscular injection of calciferol 300,000 units BPC. This will effect a cure, but even so follow-up is necessary to ensure that the response is satisfactory and that a relapse does not occur.

Reference

SEELIG M.S. (1970) Are American children still getting an excess of Vitamin D? *Clinical Pediatrics*, 9, 380.

RINGWORM OF FOOT

Ringworm between the toes is treated by benzoic acid compound ointment BPC (Whitfield's ointment).

Alternatives which are no more effective are zinc undeconate ointment BNF or 1 per cent tolnaftate cream or powder (Tinaderm).

RUBELLA

No treatment is required for rubella. The child need not be put to bed. He should return to school within three or four days of the onset of the illness.

The family doctor should remember the importance of women in early pregnancy avoiding contact with a patient suffering from rubella, or a baby born with the rubella syndrome – for he is apt to be infectious for a year after birth.

Human normal immune globulin has not proved to be effective in preventing rubella when administered to women in early pregnancy; but high titre immune globulin given very early after contact may be effective – though it may not be available in many centres. Before it is given, household or other close contact should be definite, and serological tests should demonstrate the absence of rubella antibodies in the mother's serum.

A vaccine for rubella is now available, and is given between the ages of 11 and 13.

Duration of infectivity – one day before the appearance of the rash until two days after its appearance. Quarantine is not required. Incubation period: 10–21 days.

References

ANON. (1970) Rubella vaccine. *Drug and Therapeutics Bulletin*, **8**, 59.

McDONALD J.C. & PECKHAM C.S. (1967) Gammaglobulin in prevention of rubella and congenital defects. A study of 30,000 pregnancies. *Brit. Med. J.* 3, 633.

PUBLIC HEALTH LABORTATORY SERVICE WORKING PARTY (1970) Studies of the effect of immunoglobulin on rubella in pregnancy. *Brit. Med. J.* 2, 497.

RUMINATION

Rumination is a peculiar habit whereby some babies deliberately try to bring milk up from the stomach; they arch their back, push the abdomen in and out, and bring the milk up, sometimes appearing to gargle with it. It is thought that there is usually a large element of emotional deprivation, and it follows that every effort should be made to persuade the mother to give the baby extra love and attention, picking him up when he cries for love.

It is more difficult for the baby to ruminate in the prone position. It is worth trying to keep him in that position, with the head end raised. It would be wise to refer the child to a consultant in order to ensure that the diagnosis is correct, and that the symptoms are not due to a hiatus hernia.

Reference

RICHMOND J.B., EDDY E.J. & GREEN M. (1958) Rumination, a psychosomatic syndrome of infancy. *Pediatrics*, **22**, 49.

SALIVATION (Drooling)

Some mentally defective or athetoid children, and occasional normal ones, continue to 'drool' long after normal children have learned to control their saliva. These children constantly drool over their clothes and greatly distress their mothers.

A speech therapist might be able to teach an older athetoid to control the saliva, but could not help a defective child. For such a child an atropine derivative may be the answer. One begins with a small dose of tincture of belladonna and increases it every two or three days until the mouth is sufficiently dry to stop the trouble. The correct dose must be found for each individual child. It is obvious that the greatest care must be exerted in giving this treatment, constant supervision being required. Properly carried out, the treatment earns the gratitude of the mother.

SCABIES

After a hot bath and a wash with soap, either 1 per cent gamma benzene hexachloride cream (Lorexane) is applied (once only), or 25 per cent benzoyl benzoate emulsion BNF, rubbing it in vigorously into the whole body except the face and scalp. The benzoyl benzoate is applied again 12–24 hours later, followed by a bath next day, and on the third day a change of underwear, bedclothes and blankets. Another preparation is monosulphiram 25 per cent diluted with two or three parts of water; it is applied before going to bed, covering all parts with it except the face and scalp. The infection of the clothing and bedding may be destroyed by boiling, washing in hot soap and water, or pressing with a hot iron.

It is essential to treat the whole family at the same time, even though it is not obvious that the others are also infected.

Monosulphiram 25 per cent is produced with the trade name Tetmosol, lotion or soap.

Reference

WARIN R. (1967) The treatment of scabies. *Prescribers' Journal*, 7, 14.

SCARLET FEVER

The treatment is that of acute streptococcal tonsillitis (p. 259).

SCHOOL PHOBIA

Distaste for school varies from mild expressions of dislike for school to tears on getting ready for school, or symptoms such as headache, vomiting, diarrhoea or abdominal pain, or, further, to frank and absolute refusal to go to school. It has to be distinguished from truancy, which consists of failing to go to school, nothing being said to the parents or school about it.

The treatment depends on the extent of the problem. Mere comments about dislike for school must be ignored. If the child sheds tears or develops somatic symptoms, such as vomiting or abdominal pain, the cause should be sought. This may be found in bullying, unkindness by a teacher, teasing on account of obesity or unpleasant clothes, or inability to keep up with classmates, usually in one subject such as arithmetic. If a child is particularly backward in reading, the possibility of a specific learning disorder (dyslexia) should be investigated. The doctor may consult the School Medical Officer or the head teacher. The parent may obtain the necessary guidance by a visit to the school and a discussion with the teacher. In many cases it is clear that the parents' attitude is the cause of the problem; they convey to the child by various subtle or obvious ways that they doubt whether the child will like school and settle down there, reassuring him that it will be all right, thereby suggesting that he will not like it. Another attitude which may lead to school troubles is parental overambition – expectations of achievement beyond the child's capability. Their attitude to illness may be a factor; if they keep the child away from school for every trivial symptom, the child will learn to feign symptoms, to dislike school and to seek excuses for not going, and so he will drop behind his fellows.

True school phobia, in which the child firmly refuses to go to school, is much more difficult. Iti s widely accepted that school phobia is more a fear or dislike of being separated from the mother than actual fear of school – though absence from school, a change of class, or a minor emotional upset at school, may be the trigger for the final refusal. The mother tries to insist on the child going to school, but yet makes it clear by subtle words that she would not be annoyed if he did not go.

The problem is a difficult one. The family doctor can help to wean the child away from the mother. The child should be got back to school as soon as possible, unless he is really terrified of going, in which case he will have to be kept away. Drugs will not help. The child should be referred to a paediatrician without delay; he may need the help of a child psychiatrist.

References

KAHN J.H. & NURSTEN J.P. (1968) *Unwillingly to school*. London, Pergamon.
TYERMAN M.J. (1968) *Truancy*. London, University of London Press.

SCOLIOSIS

If a child is found to have scoliosis, he should be referred to the orthopaedic consultant. Treatment is difficult if the scoliosis is not merely postural. (If it is postural, the scoliosis will disappear when the child bends over.) Structural scoliosis, if untreated, may lead to severe respiratory difficulties in early adult life.

SCURFY SCALP

A scurfy scalp in a baby, or 'cradle cap', can be treated, if mild, by washing the scalp each night with 1 per cent cetrimide lotion. More severe cases are treated by rubbing in salicylic acid 3 per cent, sulphur praecip 3 per cent in ung petrolatum for two consecutive nights.

SHYNESS

Almost all children go through phases of shyness. For instance, it is usual for the child of 12–18 months to hide behind his mother when spoken to. When an older child is excessively shy, the shyness may be due partly to inherited personality, and partly to lack of opportunity to mix with children and adults. In either case, it is important that the child should be given more opportunity to meet children and adults, and to play with children of his own age. It may be useful for the child to attend a nursery school if one is available.

It is useless to say to the child, 'Don't be shy' – as most mothers do, and it is positively harmful to ridicule the child for being shy. If the shyness is largely an inherited trait, it may help the mother to be reminded of this. The shyness should never be mentioned in the child's presence.

SLEEP REFUSAL (Insomnia)

Sleep refusal is one of the commonest behaviour problems. The majority of children present some problem connected with sleep. I have discussed the problems in detail in *The Normal Child* (Illingworth 1968). There are several factors which combine to cause sleep refusal. They are as follows.

(1) *Differences in sleep requirements.* Some children, especially the more active and the more intelligent ones, need less sleep than others. A mother becomes worried when her children sleep much less than she thinks they should.

(2) *Habit formation.* This is at the root of most problems. When the child aged 9 months or so discovers that if he howls when put to bed or on waking, he will be taken downstairs or into his mother's bed, or that his mother will come and sit and play with him, he howls every night – and often many times a night. This habit must be broken; it is much better never to start it. The child has to be left crying. It is in his own interest to obtain sufficient sleep, and certainly in his parents' interests to have an undisturbed evening and night. Indirectly the child gains from

I

the improved temper and tolerance shown by his parents if they have had an uninterrupted sleep. The mother must see that the child is safe when he cries out; she should always go to see him if he emits a sudden scream; he may have vomited, strangled himself, or had a nightmare; but she must not go to see him whenever he whimpers or cries. The doctor may help the mother by giving the child chloral for a week only, in order to break the habit; for a year-old baby I would begin with 300 mg. on the first night, half-an-hour before he is put to bed; if that proved insufficient, I would give 450 mg. the next night; and if that is insufficient, I would give 600 mg. the next night. It is never necessary to continue longer than a week; it is only given to break the habit. In order to avoid errors, it is wise to prescribe chloral in terms of mg. rather than of ml. of syrup. I do not think that dichloralphenazone (Welldorm) or trichloryl (Trichlofos) have any advantage over chloral. They are said to taste better, but I do not agree.

In my opinion it is never right to prescribe barbiturates for a child's insomnia. Phenobarbitone is almost useless. Prescribing is merely a substitute for giving time to discuss the management of the child.

It is particularly difficult for a mother if she is in her mother-in-law's house or has unkind neighbours who complain if the child cries. If she leaves him to cry, they complain; and if she tries to make him go to sleep, he stays awake.

(3) *Maternal anxiety*. Mothers keep going into the child's room to see if he is still breathing. The child then stays awake until she comes.

(4) *Lack of discipline*. This applies to the older child from three years onwards. The child is now old enough to understand that he must not disturb his parents at night or in the early morning. It is absurd to allow a school child to call out repeatedly for his parents in the evenings.

(5) *The child's love for his mother*. The child who repeatedly calls out is not being naughty; he loves his parents.

(6) *The ego and negativism*. If the child aged 1–3 can get the whole house revolving around his sleep, he will love it. Children will go to sleep if only their parents will let them; it is quite unnecessary to try to make them go to sleep.

(7) *Causes of awakening*. The child may awaken because he is too hot, too cold, has an itch, or is sharing his parents' room. He should be in his own room.

Early morning waking in a child aged 1–3 years is annoying for the parents, but there is nothing they can do about it. They may try putting him to bed earlier or later at night, but it does not make any difference.

The child should be given plenty of toys to play with when he wakes. It is not until about 3 years of age that he is old enough to understand that he must stay in his room and must not awaken his parents. Before that age there is no good answer to the problem.

Reference

ILLINGWORTH R.S. (1968) *The Normal Child: Some Problems of the First Five Years and their Treatment.* 4th edn. London, Churchill.

SNAKE BITE

The adder bite is the most common snake bite in the British Isles. It causes more anxiety, fear and discomfort than danger. The treatment consists of cleaning and then covering the bitten part and immobilizing it, applying a cold compress if possible, and giving a sedative. If the child is vomiting, he may be placed in the prone position and given chlorpromazine. An antihistamine such as promethazine (Phenergan) or chlorpheniramine (Piriton) may be given. If there is serious anxiety about an allergic response, hydrocortisone 100 mg. may be given intramuscularly. Antiserum is not advised; allergy to the horse serum is more dangerous than an adder bite.

Some advocate the use of a tourniquet at sufficient pressure to constrict the venous return without impeding arterial flow, but others think that it is unwise unless there is reason to fear a serious allergic response. A child with anything but a mild reaction should be sent to hospital.

Preparation should be given in the following doses.

Chlorpheniramine (Piriton)

1–5 years 2·5–5 ml. (2 mg. in 5 ml.) t.d.

6–12 years 3–4 tablets a day (4 mg. tablets)

Promethazine (Phenergan)

6–12 years 10–25 mg. t.d.

References

ANON. (1966) Adder bite in Britain. *Drug and Therapeutics Bulletin,* 4, 65.
ANON. (1969) Treatment of adder bite (leading article). *Brit. Med. J.* 3, 370.

SNUFFLES

Some young babies in the early weeks have a clear mucoid discharge from the nose. It clears up spontaneously, and no treatment is required. Nose drops (*e.g.* ephedrine) are unnecessary, and may damage the nasal mucosa. If the nose becomes blocked, it should be cleaned with pledgets of cotton wool.

Snuffles in the young baby is of no significance; but a purulent nasal discharge in a toddler, if unilateral, suggests a foreign body in the nose; if bilateral, it suggests an antrum infection.

SOILING (Faecal incontinence)

When a child some months or years after acquiring control of bowel emptying begins to soil, the usual cause is constipation (p. 124); but soiling may occur without constipation, in which case it is much more difficult to treat.

When soiling is due to constipation, the usual story is that there is 'diarrhoea', and that the child is constantly soiling his pants. On rectal examination it is found that there is a huge mass of solid faeces in the rectum, reaching down almost to the anus. Treatment consists of an enema or enemas to clear the rectum so that it can be re-educated. The treatment is continued with liquid paraffin.

Soiling without constipation is a troublesome behaviour problem related to insecurity, and commonly associated with urinary incontinence. No medicine will have any effect. It is necessary to try to determine the reason for the insecurity, such as domestic friction, excess scolding, troubles at school or bullying. If the family doctor finds that he is unable to determine the cause, the child should be referred to a child psychiatrist.

SORENESS AROUND THE MOUTH (Infant)

This is cured by equal parts of Lassar's paste and soft paraffin applied three or four times a day.

SPEECH, DELAYED

The commonest cause of delayed speech is mental subnormality. The next commonest cause is probably genetic – the child taking after one of his parents who was late in learning to talk. In neither of these cases is any treatment possible. Delayed speech is *not* due to the child being lazy; it is *not* due to 'everything being done for him'. Efforts to try to make the child speak will achieve nothing but harm, for they may cause troublesome behaviour problems. He does not speak because he cannot speak. Delayed speech is *not* due to tongue-tie. Delayed speech is common in twins. It is said by some that each twin understands the other's speech, and as a result does not bother to speak properly. I doubt this. It is much more likely to be due to the fact that the mother of twins has less time to talk to the children and read to them than she has to a singleton. The delay in twins may be an unexplained developmental problem.

As in the case of any normal child, the parent should read to the child, pointing out the names of objects in books, and naming common daily objects about the house and elsewhere. There is no place for speech therapy in these cases; a speech therapist cannot teach a child to talk until he is ready for it; she can only help him to speak more distinctly when he is speaking but speaking indistinctly. Part of the routine examination of any child with delayed speech is a test of hearing, including in particular high-tone deafness. Hence any child with delayed speech should be referred to a paediatrician for establishment of the diagnosis.

SPINA BIFIDA

The newborn baby found to have a meningomyelocele should be referred immediately to a paediatric surgeon, who may decide to close the meningomyelocele in the first 24 hours when there is still movement in the legs; for when the sac dries, the legs may lose all movement. A baby with a meningocele is also referred to the paediatric surgeon, but the situation is not so urgent.

The child with spina bifida will be under the care of a paediatrician or surgeon. The various problems facing the parents of an affected child are described in the booklet by Lorber (1968), and all parents of a child with spina bifida should obtain a copy. The book deals with the expression of urine, appliances for incontinence, the risk of fractures, the care of the skin and teeth, and attention to the diet. The family doctor is likely to be involved in treating urinary tract infections, and supervising the protection of the insensitive skin of paralysed legs against pressure, friction and heat. He will advise on the diet, including vitamin cover, and the prevention of obesity which is common because of inactivity.

Parents should be encouraged to join the Association for Spina Bifida whose address is given after the reference.

Reference

LORBER J. (1968) Your child with spina bifida: A practical guide to parents. Obtainable from the Association for Spina Bifida and Hydrocephalus, 112 City Road, London EC1.

SQUINT

A baby with a squint should be referred to an ophthalmologist at the age of 6 months. If a squint remains untreated after the age of about 12 months, the vision in the squinting eye may become permanently suppressed, so that the eye is blind. It is wrong to wait to see whether the child will 'grow out of it'.

STEALING

It is difficult to draw the line between the normal small child's lack of respect for the property of others and stealing. Perfectionist mothers who are determined to bring their children up to be models of virtue are apt to be worried when their child appears to be making little progress towards the absolute honesty which they demand (but do not exhibit themselves). The family doctor has to guide such mothers and persuade them not to expect too much of their children. Nevertheless, the time comes when it is fair to apply the word 'stealing' to the child's acts, and stealing is a serious matter especially when it occurs at school.

When a parent complains that her child is stealing, the first essential is to determine where the stealing occurs. If the child is stealing from the mother only, the problem is immediately localized to the mother–child relationship, and it is much easier to deal with this than with stealing at school or in shops.

The vital essential step towards treating the problem is to determine the cause of the child's feeling of insecurity, for insecurity is the basis of the problem; the child feels that he has lost his parents' love and his feeling of importance. The family doctor is in the ideal position to help because he knows the family background and knows the parents. He will know whether there is a family history of stealing. He must know what sort of example of honesty the parents are setting – and discuss it with them, if need be; and he must know about the attitudes of the parents to stealing. If there is apparent unconcern towards it, the danger of this attitude must be explained. The doctor has to look for the usual causes of insecurity – unkindness, criticism, sarcasm, perfectionism, favouritism, cruelty, rejection, constant derogation, comparisons ('You are not nearly as clever as John'), overstrictness, constant nagging and reprimands, inconsistent management, lack of discipline, overpermissiveness, leaving the child for prolonged periods, and punishment. What the child needs is love, security, a feeling of importance. Punishment will inevitably make matters worse; it will convince the child all the more that he is not loved. It is futile to give the child long sermons about his heinous sins. Love alone is the answer; and it is not enough for a parent to *feel* love; he has to *show* it. This does not mean giving the child everything that money can buy; it does not mean giving him presents; it means the facial expression, the tone of voice; it means making him feel loved, wanted, important.

247

Although the answer will be found mainly in the home, it is important to make sure that there is no discoverable cause of unhappiness at school. Bullying by a teacher or by his peers may result in the child's insecurity and in any one of a variety of behaviour problems. Judicious enquiries at the school may be useful. There is no place for medicine in dealing with this problem.

STINGS

For a bee or wasp sting, there is no specific treatment (*e.g.* the application of acid, alkali or anything else). An antihistamine cream (*e.g.* mepyramine Anthisan) or lignocaine ointment would give relief. If there is a severe allergic reaction, one would give an injection of adrenaline (*e.g.* 1 in 1,000), and chlorpheniramine (Piriton) by mouth; but normally no treatment is required.

For a jellyfish sting, the treatment is similar.

STOMATITIS

Ulcers in the mouth, whether herpetic or otherwise, do not respond well to treatment. Betamethazone lozenges or hydrocortisone lozenges BPC may be useful for aphthous ulcers, but the corticosteroid will be absorbed. They probably do little but relieve discomfort; an alternative is benzocaine compound lozenge BNF. Metronidazole tablets 200 mg. three times a day may help. Carbenoxolone preparations (*e.g.* biogastrone, bioral) have not been shown to be of value. Dequadin lozenges (dequalinium chloride) are said to be useful, but I have no experience of them.

Gentian violet should not be used because it so badly stains clothes and other objects. An older child may use a benzalkonium lozenge BNF several times a day. There is no place for systemic antibiotics for these virus infections.

Thrush stomatitis is treated by nystatin drops on the tongue.

References

ANON. (1967) Aphthous stomatitis. *Drug and Therapeutics Bulletin*, 5, 21.

ANON. (1967) New and old preparations for treating mouth ulcers. *Drug and Therapeutics Bulletin*, 5, 23.

STRIDOR

For acute stridor, see *Laryngotracheobronchitis*, p. 195.

Chronic stridor

The treatment depends on the cause. The numerous causes of persistent stridor were discussed by me in my book, *Common Symptoms of Disease in Childhood* (3rd edition, 1971). Every baby with chronic stridor should be referred to an ear, nose and throat specialist for laryngoscopy, in order to eliminate serious conditions which require treatment.

If the stridor is inspiratory only, it is usually due to benign congenital laryngeal stridor, which will cure itself by the age of 12–18 months; but not all cases are benign, and laryngoscopy should be performed to establish the diagnosis. If the stridor is both inspiratory and expiratory, the condition is likely to be serious, and reference to the specialist is essential. Conditions which may be found include webbed larynx, laryngeal polypi, angioma below the vocal cords, and a vascular ring in the thorax.

STUTTERING

I have discussed the problem of stuttering elsewhere (1970). It is normal for the child when learning to speak to repeat himself, to repeat syllables and to appear to stutter; nearly every child grows out of this, provided that the parents do nothing about it; but if they fear that he is beginning to stutter, tell him to speak clearly and distinctly, to take a big breath before he speaks, or to say it again, he is likely to become self-conscious about his speech and to stutter. The normal repetitions should be absolutely ignored.

By the fourth birthday a stuttering child should be referred to a speech therapist; but the family doctor has an important part to play, for numerous studies have referred to the tenseness in the home of the stutterer, the parental perfectionism, sometimes overstrictness, and the determined efforts to make the child speak clearly and well. It is far better for the parents to relax this attitude and to ignore the child's speech, going out of their way to increase his feeling of security and importance.

The speech therapist may adopt a commonly used method of treating the stutterer, namely timed syllabic speech. The child is taught to separate all syllables exactly equidistantly as he speaks. The method has proved successful, though relapse may occur.

References

ILLINGWORTH R.S. (1970) *Development of the Infant and Young Child: Normal and Abnormal.* 4th edn. London, Livingstone.

ANDREWS G. & HARRIS M. (1964) Syndrome of stuttering. *Clinics in Developmental Medicine*, No. 17. London, Heinemann.

STYE (Hordeolum)

A stye is a pyogenic infection, usually staphylococcal, of the sebaceous glands on the lid margin. Most styes drain spontaneously, but if a stye is causing a lot of discomfort, warm bathing for twenty minutes several times a day may give relief; occasionally the stye may be drained by pulling out the eyelash. Sulphacetamide or bacitracin neomycin ointment (Neobacrin) may be applied to the lid margin. An alternative is framycetin eye ointment BNF applied four times a day.

SUNBURN PREVENTION

When a child, for instance a fair-haired one, is particularly liable to sunburn, great care should be taken to prevent troublesome sunburn on holiday. Graduated exposure to the sun before the holiday starts may be possible. When the holiday begins, a good sunburn preparation should be applied before exposure to sun and at frequent intervals. It is too late to apply it after exposure; it is only of use as a preventive. It should not be forgotten that a child may acquire severe sunburn while sitting or playing at the seaside, even when he keeps in the shade.

Certain drugs cause photosensitivity and should therefore be avoided. They include demethylchlortetracycline (ledermycin), chlortetracycline (aureomycin), thiazide diuretics, phenothiazines, diphenhydramine, sulphonamides, ethionamide and griseofulvin.

There are so many anti-sunburn preparations on the market that it is hardly necessary to discuss the treatment here.

A benzophenone 10 per cent, as in mexenone BNF (Uvistat cream), is satisfactory; so is 15 per cent para-amino-benzoic acid in hydrous emulsifying base, which is said to have a longer-lasting effect.

Reference

Anon. (1963) Sunscreen preparations. *Drug and Therapeutics Bulletin*, 1, 17.

TALIPES

The newborn baby with talipes equinovarus should be referred to the orthopaedic surgeon during the first week after birth. He will decide whether splinting is necessary. For the so-called postural type, when the foot is of normal shape, the heel is of normal size, and the foot is mobile and can be placed in the fully over-corrected position without difficulty, no treatment is necessary; it cures itself. When in doubt, orthopaedic advice should be sought.

TEETH

Care of the teeth

Cleaning of the teeth should begin as soon as they erupt. Dental advice should be sought certainly by the second or third birthday, with particular regard to orthodontics. Overcrowding of teeth predisposes to dental caries and malocclusion spoils the appearance.

The sweet-eating habit should not be started, for this is one of the main causes of dental caries and of obesity.

Injury to the teeth with fracture or avulsion demands immediate treatment by an expert dentist. The broken part must be preserved, for reimplantation may well succeed.

Some babies are born with a tooth. The tooth is usually loose because of poor root formation, but it is better not to remove it in fear of inhalation, because of the risk of bleeding (from the physiological hypoprothrombinaemia in the newborn period) and the possibility of malposition of succeeding teeth which might result. The root soon forms so that the tooth becomes securely fixed.

There is considerable variation in the age at which the first teeth erupt. No treatment is available for delayed dentition.

TEETHING

Most of the symptoms ascribed to teething are not due to teething at all; for instance, crying in the evening is far more likely to be due to bad habit formation, the child having discovered that if he cries out he will be taken downstairs and played with, or taken into his mother's bed.

It is rarely necessary to prescribe any medicine or local application for teething.

Seward (1969) showed by means of a double blind trial that an application of lignocaine hydrochloride, benzyl alcohol, tincture of myrrh in menthol, honey, sorbic acid and SVR 90 per cent alcohol, was highly effective.

Lignocaine hydrochloride	0·3 per cent
Benzyl alcohol	0·3 per cent
Tinct myrrh	0·8 per cent
Menthol	0·06 per cent
Honey	20·0 per cent
Sorbic acid	0·1 per cent
SVR BP 90 per cent alcohol	3·0 per cent
Sweetened flavoured aqueous base to	100·0 per cent

Put three drops on a clean finger tip and massage gently into the gum; if necessary, repeat in 15–20 minutes.

If a sedative has to be given, which is not unusual, chloral is safe. An alternative is aspirin.

My opinion is that no treatment is necessary.

Reference

SEWARD M.H. (1969) The effectiveness of a teething solution in infants. *British Dental Journal*, 127, 457.

TEMPER TANTRUMS

Most children have at least one temper tantrum. If they discover that by throwing a vigorous temper tantrum they can attract attention, cause consternation and anxiety, or better still get their own way, they will soon realize that the energy and effort required are well worth while, and the tantrums will continue. The immediate treatment is to ignore them as far as possible, and on no account to let the child have his own way by having a tantrum. The mother should go into another room, closing the door, leaving the child lying on his back screaming and kicking. It is most disappointing for a child to have a temper tantrum ignored by his uninterested mother.

It is important to prevent tantrums by dealing with any source of insecurity, such as friction in the home, overstrictness, constant reprimands or favouritism to another child. It must also be remembered that hunger, causing hypoglycaemia, may be at the root of bad temper, especially in children returning from school. The treatment in this case is to supply food as quickly as possible and not to argue with the child or reprimand him or give him a sermon.

TESTIS, TORSION OF

Torsion of the testis is an acute emergency demanding immediate and correct treatment. The symptoms are likely to be crying and vomiting.

The pain may be localized to the scrotum or to the iliac fossa. The immediate treatment is to rotate the testis in the opposite direction. The correct direction is easily determined; if one attempts to rotate it in the wrong direction, pain will be increased; it is eased by 'derotation'. The child is then immediately referred to the paediatric surgeon so that a recurrence is prevented.

The condition commonly resembles and is confused with acute epididymo-orchitis.

Reference

SPARKS J.P. (1970) Torsion of the testis. *Practitioner*, 205, 191.

TESTES, UNDESCENDED

If a testis can be pushed into the scrotum, it is a retractile testis, and no treatment is required.

There has been a difference of opinion about the age at which undescended testes should be operated upon. The tendency has been to operate earlier than formerly, on the ground that fertility is more likely if operation is performed early. It is commonly advised now that the operation should be performed at the age of about 4, before starting school.

There is no place for hormonal treatment. Apart from being useless, it carries risks, including that of sterility.

THRIVE, FAILURE TO

The numerous causes of failure to thrive are discussed in *Common Symptoms of Disease in Children* (Illingworth 1971). The treatment must depend on the cause. In essence, the causes can be summarized as follows.

(1) Defective intake
(2) Defective absorption – fat, carbohydrate, protein.

(3) Defective metabolism – renal acidosis, hypercalcaemia, nephrogenic diabetes insipidus, etc.

(4) Severe disease of the brain (*e.g.* mental deficiency), heart (congenital), chest (asthma, bronchiectasis), pancreas (diabetes, fibrocystic disease), liver (cirrhosis), kidney (chronic renal insufficiency), chronic infection.

(5) Increased loss – diarrhoea, vomiting.

Before becoming involved in numerous investigations, it is essential to eliminate the first group, defective intake. Many mothers claim that they are giving the child all that he needs in nourishing food, whereas in fact the child is starving. The family doctor is in a better position than anyone to diagnose this and treat it.

The more important of the remaining conditions have been discussed elsewhere in this book.

The most common cause of a well child being unusually small for his age is the simple fact that he takes after his mother or father.

THRUSH

Oral thrush. Drops of nystatin 1 ml. 100,000 units are placed four times a day on to the tongue. No attempt is made to remove the thrush lesions.

Gentian violet should not be used because it stains clothes and other objects.

Thrush nappy rash. This usually clears with nystatin ointment applied four times a day. If the thrush is secondary to ammonia dermatitis, that should be treated (p. 206).

An alternative treatment for dermal thrush is amphotericin B (fungilin) 3 per cent cream or 3 per cent ointment applied three times a day.

Vaginal thrush is treated by candeptin vaginal ointment

THUMBSUCKING

All babies suck their thumbs, fingers or wrist, some in utero, and some more than others. No treatment is required, as it is a harmless occupation, provided only that it stops by the age of 6 years, as it nearly always does. If it continues after the age of 6 years, it will cause deformity of the front teeth in about 1 in 8 children. Thumbsucking may cause some soreness of the digits and even thickening of the skin, but it is not of importance. Determined efforts to make a child stop sucking his fingers will cause it to continue as an attention-seeking device. The habit should be ignored.

TICS

There is no satisfactory treatment for tics. No medicine makes any difference. It is wrong to prescribe barbiturates or, worse still, tranquillizing drugs, because of their ineffectiveness for the purpose and their side effects.

Tics are annoying to parents, and it is important that they should not express their annoyance, reprimanding the child for the tics. After all, the movements are not deliberate, and arise from the subconscious mind. Reprimands are apt to increase underlying insecurity and to make the child self-conscious about the tics, with the result that they continue. The tics should not be discussed in the child's presence.

In my experience it is unusual to be able to find any faults in management or worries at school the treatment of which stops the tics. Tics usually, but not always, disappear spontaneously; parental efforts to stop them by reprimands will make them worse.

TINEA CAPITIS

Tinea capitis is cured in one or two months by griseofulvin given in the following doses:
Up to 1 year: 62·5 mg. b.d. for 7–10 days,
1–5 years: 62·5 mg. t.d. for 7–10 days,
6–12 years: 125 mg. b.d. or t.d. for 7–10 days.
    Tablets contain 125 mg.

TOES, CURLY

When one toe lies on top of or under another, strapping rarely helps. There will be no trouble until shoes are worn, when surgical treatment may be required. If they are merely curly without overlapping, they should be left untreated. The development of soreness is an indication for operation.

TOEING-IN

According to my orthopaedic colleague, W.J.W. Sharrard, in-toeing is nearly always a hip deformity due to natural changes in the plane of the acetabulum and the angle of anteversion of the neck of the femur during the first five or six years of life. There is no specific treatment which has any effect, except that sometimes it is associated with pes planovalgus which in itself may require shoe alteration; this can be judged by inspection of the shoe. The condition cures itself.

Occasionally in-toeing persists beyond the age of 6 or 7 years, or even begins to develop at that age as a familial feature. This rarely corrects itself, and calls for a rotation osteotomy of the femur in later childhood.

TONGUE-TIE

It is never necessary to operate for tongue-tie in the first year, and it is doubtful whether any operation is needed after that. Tongue-tie will never delay speech, and many speech experts consider that it cannot even cause indistinct speech. I have never seen a child in which tongue-tie interfered with sucking and feeding.

If there is marked tongue-tie with a depression in the front part of the surface of the tongue, so that it will be difficult for the child to protrude the tongue, the operation may be considered by the age of about 2 years. I doubt whether the operation is ever necessary, but if it is done, it should be done by a plastic or paediatric surgeon, and never by the family doctor, because of the risk of haemorrhage.

TONSILLECTOMY

It is said that in the United States tonsillectomy costs $150 m. a year and 300 deaths. In 1954 it was estimated that in England and Wales the cost of tonsillectomy was about £3m.

In 1961 I reviewed the indications for tonsillectomy, and research since then in various parts of the world has done nothing to make me alter the views then expressed. I wrote that neither tonsillectomy nor any other operation should be performed on a child because the parents, aunt, mother-in-law or school nurse wish it; the child alone matters, and no operation should be performed unless it is in his interests. Tonsils should not be removed on account of mere size, unless they are so large that they are causing respiratory obstruction. This is rare. Recent work has shown that respiratory obstruction due to tonsils may cause cor pulmonale; but unless the tonsils are so large that they are virtually meeting in the midline, this risk does not occur. Apart from this, the size is irrelevant. It is quite wrong to think that large tonsils are more likely to be associated with recurrent infections than small tonsils, or that large tonsils are more likely to be infected than small ones. It must be remembered that it is normal for a 5- or 6-year-old to have large tonsils, and that these tonsils become smaller in size as the child gets older.

Tonsils should never be removed because of frequent colds. It has been shown repeatedly that tonsillectomy does not reduce the frequency of colds.

The idea of focal sepsis was discarded many years ago. Tonsils should never be removed for any general disease, such as rheumatic fever, rheumatoid arthritis or asthma.

Tonsils should not be removed because they 'look infected'. Apart from acute tonsillitis, there is no relationship between the appearance of the tonsils and the symptoms which they cause (except only in the case of the rare gross enlargement mentioned above – when the symptom of obstruction is related to the size).

Tonsils should not be removed for frequent tonsillitis unless continuous prophylactic penicillin (200,000 units of penicillin G twice a day, or 250 mg. phenoxymethyl penicillin twice a day) for several months has failed to prevent frequent acute tonsillitis with fever.

I suggest that tonsils should be removed if a child has three or four attacks of acute tonsillitis with fever per year in spite of continuous prophylactic penicillin; that they should be removed for gross obstruction, or after a peritonsillar abscess. There are no other indications. Adenoidectomy is a completely different problem, which has been discussed on p. 79.

Before suggestions that a child should have the tonsils removed, one should be fully aware of the possible complications. Some 280 articles on the subject of these complications were listed in the *Quarterly Cumulative Index Medicus* over a 10-year period. In the USA the operation is said to cause more deaths than diphtheria, rubella, scarlet fever, chickenpox and whooping cough combined. There is always a risk in an anaesthetic; the risk of cardiac arrest under anaesthesia has been put at 1 in 2,300. Other complications are haemorrhage, otitis media, antrum infection, acute nephritis, inhalation of septic material, displacement or knocking out of teeth, and psychological disturbances such as enuresis.

References

BOLANDE R.P. (1969) Ritualistic surgery – circumcision and tonsillectomy. *New Engl. J. Med.* **280**, 591.

ILLINGWORTH R.S. (1961) The tonsillectomy problem. *Proc. Roy. Soc. Med.* **54**, 393.

MACARTNEY F.J., PANDAY J. & SCOTT O. (1969) Cor pulmonale as a result of chronic nasopharyngeal obstruction due to hypertrophied tonsils and adenoids. *Arch. Dis. Childh.* **44**, 585.

TONSILLITIS

There is a difference between what is ideal and what is practical. Ideally, when a child is found to have acute tonsillitis or an acutely inflamed sore throat, and it is thought not to be merely the beginning of a cold, a throat swab should be taken. If next day streptococci have been cultured, the infection should be treated immediately with penicillin – largely with the aim of preventing rheumatic fever or acute nephritis, but also with the knowledge that proper treatment will cause a rapid cure and disappearance of the offending organisms.

In practice, it is not always possible to obtain a throat swab report the day after the swab has been taken. In that case one has to treat the tonsillitis as if it is streptococcal, discontinuing the penicillin if the swab is negative.

If the parents cannot be relied upon to give phenoxymethyl penicillin 6-hourly day and night, I would commence treatment with an injection of triplopen, and next day commence oral therapy. This should be continued for ten days, for it has been shown that if the penicillin is discontinued sooner, the streptococci are commonly not eradicated.

It is hardly ever necessary to prescribe a gargle; gargles have no effect on the tonsillitis, but a gargle containing phenol (*e.g.* phenol gargle BPC) may have a soothing effect if the child complains of severe soreness of the throat.

TOOTH SOCKET, BLEEDING

The mouth should be washed out, blood clots being removed by a swab. A gauze roll is then placed in the socket, and kept in place by biting it for at least five minutes. The patient must not at intervals release the clench in order to determine whether bleeding is continuing. The jaws should be kept clenched well past the normal clotting time. The swab may be infiltrated with 2 per cent local anaesthetic containing 1 in 100,000 parts of adrenaline.

If necessary, the gingivae are injected with a local anaesthetic on each side of the socket and the gum is sutured to close the bleeding point.

Reference

James P., Prasad S.V.L. & Fisher A.D. (1970) The bleeding tooth socket. *Brit. J. Hosp. Med.* 3, 359.

TORTICOLLIS

Congenital torticollis, associated with a sternomastoid tumour, is treated by the mother. She twists the baby's head round in both directions many times a day, until the torticollis has disappeared. Only if it persists beyond the age of 6–9 months should the child be referred to the paediatric surgeon for operation on the sternomastoid muscle; if allowed to persist, the torticollis becomes associated with facial asymmetry.

Acute torticollis may be due to cervical adenitis or other inflammatory condition in the neck. Chronic torticollis may be of ocular origin and the opinion of the appropriate specialist should be sought.

TRAVEL ABROAD

Although this subject is not strictly relevant to the treatment of the child in the home, this book is intended for the family doctor, and the family doctor is likely to have to advise parents about precautions to be taken when about to travel abroad with their children. Accordingly I decided to include a brief note about the matter.

Some countries have reciprocal National Health arrangements with this country; they are Norway, Sweden, Denmark, Yugoslavia and Bulgaria. Cover does not extend to pre-existing conditions. In any case it is essential when travelling abroad to have really adequate insurance, which also allows one parent to come back home sooner than the other. For this purpose each parent should have all the children's names on his or her passport. Wherever possible, prompt return home by air should be the aim for anything but an acute illness; it certainly would be for a fracture after the initial emergency treatment.

Many countries require a certificate of smallpox vaccination; this is valid for three years.

Other immunization may be required. TAB immunization is recommended for a visit to Spain, and certainly for the North African coast.

If a child is to visit an area where infective hepatitis is prevalent, he may be protected by gammaglobulin 0·04 ml./lb.; this gives protection for four months.

Equipment

This should include bandages, gauze, steristrip, cotton wool, strapping, eye drops, salt tablets, sun-glasses, splinter forceps, thermometer, waterproof dunbell dressings; a Kepcool or Insulex insulated bag for picnics; tins of milk and lemonade powder; large Thermos flasks; polythene water containers; a Bluet or similar heater for boiling water if going to Spain; and possibly chlorine water sterilizing tablets (Halazane).

Medicine taken would include ampicillin, aspirin, antidiarrhoea medicine containing tinct opii, and diphenoxylate; and a zinc and castor oil ointment.

Insect repellants such as dimethylphthalate or diethyl toluamide are useful; the eyes and mouth should be avoided when using them. Boots Flypel is a convenient preparation. Aerosol insecticides including dicophane (DDT), gammexane or pyrethrum are also useful. Dicophane dusting powder for the prevention of bug and other insect bites may prevent troublesome urticaria.

Diarrhoea prevention

The main principle is the absolute avoidance (in countries such as Spain, or elsewhere if hygiene is poor) of unboiled water (even for brushing the teeth), unboiled milk, ice-creams, salads, unskinned fruits, cream cakes, shellfish, prepared or cold meats. This does not apply to Switzerland, Northern Italy, France or Scandinavia, where there is no greater risk of infection than in this country. It is said that one chlorine tablet (Halazine) per litre of water after shaking and allowing to stand for thirty minutes is effective for sterilizing it.

When visiting a country where diarrhoea is prevalent (*e.g.* Spain), there is much to be said for prophylactic 'streptotriad' – streptomycin and sulphonamides; the tablet contains streptomycin 65 mg., sulphadiazine 100 mg., sulphadimidine 100 mg., and sulphathiazole 100 mg. At 7 years half a tablet is given three times a day, and at 12 years 1 tablet three times a day. At 3 years one gives half a 5 ml. spoonful of the suspension twice a day. Clioquinol (Enterovioform) is probably of no value and may have serious neurological side effects.

Sunburn prevention

See p. 250.

Heat exhaustion

Salt tablets should be used. The symptoms are lethargy, vertigo, headache, vomiting and collapse.

Heatstroke

The child is stripped and sprayed continuously with cold water, with an electric fan directed towards him.

Preparation

Chalk and opium mixture BNF 1–5 years 2–5 ml.

References

ILLINGWORTH R.S. (1969) Taking children abroad. *Community Health*, 1, 112.
SMITH R.N. (1969) Medical treatment on holiday abroad. *Brit. Med. J.* 2, 303.

TRAVEL SICKNESS

The most effective drug for the prevention of travel sickness is hyoscine. It can be given conveniently in the form of Kwells (0·3 mg. hyoscine per tab.), $\frac{1}{4}$–$\frac{1}{2}$ a tablet at the age of 3–7 years, $\frac{1}{2}$–1 tablet at 7 years and over. For an adolescent, 2 tablets may be given. In each case the drug should be given half-an-hour before the journey. If at sea, a dose should be given half-an-hour before rising from the bed. The maximum dose in 24 hours is $1\frac{1}{2}$ tablets under the age of 7, and 3 tablets in 24 hours over 7 years. The drug has a cumulative effect and should be discontinued as soon as possible.

Antihistamine drugs, *e.g.* meclizine (Ancolan) (the longest acting), mepyramine maleate (Anthisan) are of some value. They tend to cause drowsiness, which may be of advantage.

Preparations

Meclizine – age 6–12 years 12·5 mg. 6-hourly.

Mepyramine

elixir 1–5 years 5–10 ml. (25 mg. in 5 ml.)
tablets age 6–12 years 50 mg.

Reference

WADE O.L. & DUNDEE J.W. (1969) Antiemetic drugs. *Prescribers' Journal*, 2, 69.

TUBERCULOSIS

Over the age of 2 years, there is no need to prescribe treatment for primary tuberculosis; below that age, treatment with isoniazid and PAS is given for six months. In any case periodical chest X-rays are essential in order to check that healing is satisfactory.

There is no need to confine a child with primary tuberculosis to bed, or to isolate him from others, or to send him to a sanatorium. In Sheffield my colleagues treated many hundreds of children with primary tuberculosis, and always allowed then normal activity. They were all followed up over a prolonged period, and the results were excellent. Even children with miliary or meningeal tuberculosis are allowed up and about in hospital as soon as they feel fit to be up (Lorber 1956). Extensive studies in France and elsewhere showed that there is virtually no risk of infection by a child with primary tuberculosis.

Drugs for tuberculosis have been reviewed in the papers mentioned below. They include isoniazid, streptomycin, para-amino-salicylic acid and rifampicin. The latter must be used with other drugs, for rapid resistance develops; it is expensive, treatment costing about £200 per year. Ethambutol is another expensive drug, costing £100 for a year's treatment. Other drugs include capreomycin, ethionamide, cycloserine, kanamycin, viomycin and pyrazinamide. All these drugs are toxic. None of them would be prescribed by the family doctor. Many of them have important side effects, and an affected child would be under the care of a chest physician.

The prevention of tuberculosis by BCG is discussed on p. 44. The family doctor plays an important part in prevention by seeing that any child who is a contact of tuberculosis is given BCG, even though the contact's infection is said to have completely healed.

References

ANON. (1968) Todays' drugs (Review). *Brit. Med. J.* 3, 664.
ANON. (1968) Drug for tuberculosis (Annotation). *Brit. Med. J.* 3, 664.
ANON. (1969) Chemotherapy of drug resistant tuberculosis (leading article). *Brit Med. J.* 3, 487.
ANON. (1969) Rifampicin (leading article). *Brit. Med. J.* 3, 487.
ANON. (1970) Rifampicin. *Drug and Therapeutics Bulletin*, 8, 11.
LORBER J. (1956) Current results of treatment of tuberculous meningitis and miliary tuberculosis. *Brit. Med. J.* 1, 1009.

ULCER, PEPTIC

Though peptic ulcer is regarded as uncommon in childhood, many adults with peptic ulcer claim that their symptoms began in childhood. The diagnosis of peptic ulcer in a child would be made by barium meal and occult blood tests, and the treatment described below would be prescribed only if the diagnosis was established radiologically.

There is no place for rest in bed for an ulcer. If the child is smoking, this should be stopped. For pain, aluminium hydroxide gel is effective. Sodium bicarbonate is effective but may cause alkalosis. Magnesium carbonate is effective but has laxative properties. Magnesium trisilicate is less effective and bismuth even less so.

The diet should be a normal one except for foods which cause ulcer pain. Snacks may abolish hunger pains. Special diets are no more effective than a normal diet.

Carbenoxolone, a synthetic derivative of liquorice, may be of value in the treatment of peptic ulcer.

Preparations

Aluminium hydroxide gel (Aludrox)
BNF 1 year: 1 ml. t.d. or q.d.
        7 years: 2·5 ml. t.d. or q.d.

Magnesium carbonate mixture BPC 5 ml. t.d.

Carbenoxolone (Biogastrone) 50 mg. tablet t.d. p.c.

References

ANON. (1964) Antacids for peptic ulcer. *Drug and Therapeutics Bulletin*, 2, 6.
ANON. (1967) Diet for peptic ulcer. *Drug and Therapeutics Bulletin*, 5, 5.

ULCERATIVE COLITIS

This is a serious and difficult disease, the management and supervision of which should be in the hands of a paediatrician, who in turn will seek the advice of a surgeon and maybe a child psychiatrist. The paediatrician and surgeon between them must decide how long purely medical treatment should continue before surgery has to be embarked upon. Many children can be maintained symptom-free on medical treatment; but recourse to surgery should not be delayed if progress is unsatisfactory.

The diagnosis of ulcerative colitis must be established by sigmoido-scopy and possibly by barium enema. In the acute stage the ill child will be treated in hospital, but after that he will be under the care of the family doctor. Many children are not ill with ulcerative colitis; for these, admission to hospital is unnecessary.

There is no need for the child to be confined to bed, except in the acute stage when he prefers to be at rest.

There is no indication for a 'roughage-free' diet. It would be difficult indeed to understand the mechanism whereby a normal diet would cause more peristalsis and therefore more diarrhoea than a 'roughage-free' diet. Modern paediatric texts now no longer advocate a roughage-free diet for ulcerative colitis. It has been suggested that some adults with ulcerative colitis have fewer symptoms if they are given a milk-free diet. The rationale of this lies in the possibility that some cases are associated with allergy to cow's milk protein.

It is reasonable to supply a diet with a higher than usual calorie content, and perhaps higher protein content, in order to try to prevent or alleviate malnutrition.

Every effort should be made to correct or prevent dehydration. There may be psychological factors in patients with ulcerative colitis, but it is not easy to determine whether the psychological features of sufferers from ulcerative colitis are the cause or the result of the condition. One should certainly try to reduce anxiety and tenseness by a sedative, if necessary (*e.g.* sodium amytal). Overprotection should be avoided and the patient should be treated as far as possible as a normal child.

The drug of choice for the prevention of exacerbations of ulcerative colitis and to some extent for treatment is sulphasalazine. It may be necessary to continue with this for years, every attempt to discontinue the drug being promptly followed by the recurrence of symptoms. Like any of the sulphonamides, sulphasalazine may depress the bone marrow, and regular white cell counts (*e.g.* monthly at first, and later 3-monthly) are advisable. For the acutely ill child, hydrocortisone enemas may be needed for a few days, but such a child would be in hospital. I doubt whether there is any place for the use of corticosteroids for the treatment of a child with ulcerative colitis in general practice.

It is reasonable to prescribe diphenoxylate (Lomotil) if there is diarrhoea in spite of the sulphasalazine, and an antispasmodic drug such as propantheline bromide (Probanthine) if there is abdominal pain. Ferrous sulphate would be given if there were anaemia from malnutrition or blood loss. Multivitamin tablets would be advisable for a child with chronic diarrhoea.

A child who fails to respond to the above medical treatment should be seen by a surgeon, who may consider that radical surgery in the way of excision of the entire ulcerated portion of colon is advisable.

Preparations

Sulphasalazine (Salazopyrine) 500 mg. tablets
age 6–12 years: 0·25–1·0 g. t.d. or q.d.

1 year:	250 mg. q.d.
7 years:	500 mg. q.d.
Puberty:	1 g. q.d.

Propantheline bromide (Probanthine) 15 mg. tablets;
age 7 years 7·5 mg. t.d.

UMBILICUS

An umbilical hernia is best left untreated (see p. 188).

Umbilical sepsis in the newborn is treated by cleaning with spirit four times a day and applying chlorhexidine lotion or powder.

Umbilical granulation tissue (pyogenic granuloma) may be either left alone, apart from treatment of the infection, or touched with a silver nitrate stick; the appearance may have been modified by talcum powder, forming a flat reddish nodule (talc granuloma).

An umbilical polyp if it is bright red, or any polyp on a stalk, should not be dealt with in the home. A bright red polyp may be a relic of the omphalomesenteric duct, in which case it consists of intestinal mucosa, and should be treated by a paediatric surgeon. If there is any sign of a discharge, such as urine, the child should likewise be referred to the surgeon; it may be a relic of the urachus.

The diagnosis of umbilical conditions may not be easy. When in doubt, it would be wise to consult a paediatrician or paediatric surgeon.

URINARY TRACT INFECTION

The first essential for the treatment of a urinary tract infection is a correct diagnosis. This is a matter of considerable difficulty, and is impossible without laboratory help. It calls for microscopy of the deposit from a clean specimen of urine, culture with a total viable count and determination of the sensitivity of the organism to various antibiotics. As every hospital with a trained personnel has difficulty in obtaining a really clean specimen from a child, especially a girl, and especially when a bag has to be attached to the infant in order to obtain a specimen, it is even more difficult for a family doctor to obtain a clean specimen in a sterile jar and to take it immediately to a laboratory for examination. The hospital specialist usually has a second and often a third specimen examined in order to be sure of the diagnosis, and some specialists when still in doubt perform a bladder puncture in order to be sure that the specimen obtained is uncontaminated. Experiments are now being carried out with a dip slide ('uricult') – a microscope slide covered with culture medium; a specimen, midstream if possible, is passed onto the slide, which is immediately put into a sterile bottle and taken immediately to the laboratory for culture. Experiments are also being performed with a chemical test for bacteriuria.

When the laboratory report is received, it has to be interpreted. The paediatrician will almost invariably repeat the specimen, and frequently will obtain several specimens before he is satisfied with the diagnosis. Treatment is prolonged, and investigation of the urinary tract is carried out in all cases. Hence every child with suspected urinary tract infection should be seen by a paediatrician before antibiotic treatment is given; if an antibiotic is prescribed, the paediatrician will be uncertain of the diagnosis and may find it difficult or impossible to confirm it. He will not wish to expose the child to X-rays unless he is satisfied that the diagnosis is correct.

It is impossible to make the diagnosis on the basis of symptoms. Most children with a urinary tract infection have no urinary symptoms; and the commonest cause of dysuria in an infant or toddler is not a urinary tract infection, but a nappy rash. Apparent frequency in a toddler is commonly nothing more than an attention-seeking device. In at least half of all cases of urinary tract infection there is no albuminuria; chemical tests for albumin and pus are useless for establishing the diagnosis. In my experience the majority of children treated at home for a urinary tract infection have no such infection, whereas the diagnosis of a urinary tract infection has not usually been suspected in cases later proved to have the infection.

A variety of drugs are available for treatment. Sulphadimidine, the cheapest of all, is useful for most cases, as the common infective agent, *E. coli*, is usually sensitive to it. There is no advantage in the more expensive sulphonamides, sulphamethizole (Urolucosil) or sulphafurazole (Gantrisin). Other drugs include nitrofurantoin, nalidixic acid, trimethoprim (for gram negative organisms except pseudomonas), ampicillin (for proteus), polymixin or colistin (for pseudomonas), kanamycin, cephalexin, streptomycin and gentamicin. Mandelamine is never used for acute infections or infections by proteus or pseudomonas; it is only effective when the urine is sufficiently acidified (*e.g.* by ascorbic acid 4 g. per day); it is unlikely to cure a chronic infection but may reduce the bacterial count. Potassium citrate by itself is useless for the treatment of urinary tract infections, but it may enhance the effect of sulphonamides, kanamycin or gentamicin. For most children, sulphadimidine is entirely satisfactory. There is no justification for the routine use of the other drugs, all of which are more expensive, some (*e.g.* nalidixic acid, trimethoprim) considerably so. They should be used only when bacteriological studies indicate that their use is essential.

If there is cystitis with strangury, which would be very unusual, phenylazopyridine (pyridium) may give rapid relief of the symptoms, but it does not cure the infection. The appropriate antibiotic must also be given.

There is no need for the child to be kept in bed, unless he wants to be in bed because of a high temperature.

The duration of treatment is a matter of disagreement amongst paediatricians. Few paediatricians treat an acute case in the first attack for less than six weeks; for a chronic or second attack treatment will be for at least six months. Whatever the duration of treatment, repeated examinations of the urine with culture and total viable counts are essential. A week and a month after discontinuing treatment, and thereafter at infrequent intervals for at least two years, the urine is re-examined by the hospital laboratory.

In all cases, even in their first attack, urinary tract examination by pyelography and micturating cystourethrograms are carried out in order that appropriate treatment can be given.

Urinary tract infection in childhood is a major cause of renal failure and hypertension in adult life, and proper treatment and follow-up is essential. From what has been said above it follows that all children with suspected urinary tract infection should be referred to a paediatrician.

Preparations

	1-11 mths.	1 year	7 years	Puberty
Nalidixic acid (Negram) 500 mg. tablets: suspension 60 mg. in 1 ml.	25 mg./kg. q.d.	250 mg. q.d.	500 mg. q.d.	1 g. q.d.
Nitrofurantoin (Furadantin, Berkfurin) should be prescribed under the official name, as it is cheaper	2·5 mg./kg./q.d.	25 mg. q.d.	50 mg. q.d.	100 mg.

	1–11 mths.	*1 year*	*7 years*	*Puberty*
Sulphadimidine – avoid in the newborn period	25 mg./kg./q.d.	250 mg. q.d.	500 mg. q.d.	1 g. q.d.
Trimethoprim with sulphamethoxazole (Septrin)	20 mg. b.d.	40 mg. b.d.	80 mg. b.d.	160 mg. b.d.

Phenylazopyridine (Pyridium) 1 tablet t.d. for older child.

Reference

TAITZ L. (1971) Urinary tract infection in childhood. *Prescribers' Journal.* In Press.

URTICARIA

The treatment of urticaria depends on the cause, and there are many possible causes, including drugs and allergy to foodstuffs. The usual cause of chronic papular urticaria in a child is sensitivity to insect bites, such as fleas or bed bugs. Animals should be treated by an appropriate dusting powder, *e.g.* dicophane (DDT) for a dog and pyrethrum for a cat. The child's clothes are dusted with 10 per cent dicophane powder. The rest of the family should be disinfected if necessary. The animals' quarters are sprayed with 5 per cent DDT in kerosene. For bed bugs, the floor coverings, floorboards, skirting and furniture are sprayed with the same material.

Promethazine (Phenergan) may reduce the itching, and is of value at night because of its sedative action. The local application of 1 per cent phenol in calamine lotion may reduce the itching, or calamine liniment in 0·25 per cent menthol.

An antihistamine – diphenhydramine or chlorpheniramine, is useful in the acute stage. Aspirin may aggravate urticaria.

Preparations

Promethazine (Phergan)

age 1:   5 mg. t.d.

age 7:   10 mg. t.d.

Puberty: 25 mg. t.d.

Diphenhydramine

age 1:   12·5 mg. t.d.

age 7:   25 mg. t.d.

Puberty: 50 mg. t.d.

Chlorpheniramine (Piriton)

age 1:   1 mg. t.d.

age 7:   2 mg. t.d.

Puberty: 4 mg. t.d.

VOMITING

The causes of vomiting are so numerous that it is impossible to describe the treatment of each one here. It is obvious that treatment must depend on the cause. For cyclical vomiting see migraine (p. 201).

Whatever the cause, it is rarely necessary to prescribe an antiemetic drug such as chlorpromazine (Largactil) or prochlorperazine (Stemetil). These drugs may have serious side effects, such as oculogyric crises, even after two or three doses, and they are better avoided unless there is a good reason for prescribing them.

Preparations

Chlorpromazine 1 mg./kg./q.d.

Prochlorperazine (5 mg. tablets) syrup 5 mg. in 5 ml.

1 year: 1·25 mg. t.d.

7 years: 2·5 mg. t.d.

VULVOVAGINITIS

A clear mucoid discharge from the vagina of the newborn baby is normal. There may be some blood in the discharge from about the fifth to the tenth day, and this too is normal. A clear mucoid discharge at about the time of puberty is normal, and no treatment is required, though the girl and her mother need reassurance.

A mild vulvovaginitis may respond to simple hygiene, washing the affected parts daily, and taking care that after defaecation the girl cleans herself in the direction from the vulva to the anus, and not vice versa.

A purulent or offensive vaginal discharge usually responds to an antibiotic such as penicillin systemically. Soreness of the vulva may be treated by a silicone barrier cream.

The family doctor should always remember the possibility that there is a foreign body in the vagina. Hence if a child does not respond rapidly to the above measures she should be referred to a paediatrician for advice. The specialist will take a swab for culture and examine, if necessary, for a foreign body by means of a speculum (and perhaps an X-ray for an opaque object). If the family doctor suspects that the vulvovaginitis is gonococcal, he will seek the advice of a specialist before administering an antibiotic.

Other causes of vulvovaginitis include monilia and trichomonas. Monilia is treated by nystatin ointment or candeptin, and trichomonas by metronidazole (by mouth if the child weighs over 100 lb.; otherwise it is used locally).

Sometimes a mild vulvovaginitis responds well to an oestrogen cream which cornifies the epithelium.

WARTS

A plantar wart may be treated by a ring pad or an occlusive strip of elastoplast. If this does not cure it, a 40 per cent salicylic acid plaster for 48 hours should suffice. Foot baths of 3 per cent formalin for 30 minutes every night cure 80 per cent in 6–8 weeks. Others apply 10 per cent salicylic acid in soft paraffin or salicylic acid collodion BPC. Excision by curettage

K

after local infiltration with an anaesthetic should be carried out only as a last resort.

For filiform warts on the face or scalp or small warts on the hands or knees, the application of liquid nitrogen or a phenol stick is satisfactory.

WHEEZING

See *Asthma*.

WHOOPING COUGH

The treatment of whooping cough is unsatisfactory, but fortunately severe attacks are now rare. If there is troublesome vomiting, small frequent feeds should be given, and if vomiting occurs immediately after a feed, the feed may be repeated. It may help a child to sleep in the prone position. It is important to ensure adequate hydration. Moderate sedation with phenobarbitone may be advisable. There is no need to keep the child in bed.

Cough suppressants are contraindicated because failure to cough up thick tenaceous sputum predisposes to atelectasis. It is doubtful whether any expectorant is worth giving; it might be justifiable to give potassium iodide in order to attempt to liquefy secretions, but it should be discontinued in two or three weeks.

Antibiotics are of doubtful value. A Medical Research Council trial of chloramphenicol and chlortetracycline against an inert substance (1953) showed that chloramphenicol and chlortetracycline had a slight beneficial effect only if given within eight days of the onset of symptoms; later than that there was no significant effect. (I would not prescribe chloramphenicol because of the dangerous side effects.) Adasek *et al.* (1969) showed that neither ampicillin nor tetracycline alone or in combination shortened the duration of infectivity. Shirkey (1968) regarded ampicillin as being the drug of choice, but of doubtful efficacy (75–100 mg./kg./ day). Bass *et al.* (1969) compared treatment with ampicillin, oxytetracycline, chloramphenicol and erythromycin with no antibiotic treatment, and found that none of the antibiotics altered the clinical course. The longer the symptoms have occurred before the institution of treatment, the less likely it is that antibiotics will help. The unsatisfactory response to antibiotics may well be due to the recent observation that many cases of typical whooping cough are due to adenovirus infections and not B. Pertussis or parapertussis. Whooping cough is a condition for which large amounts of medicine are prescribed to little purpose. There is no indication for the use of atropine methyl nitrate (eumydrine), and it might do harm by drying the secretions.

It is possible that hyperimmune gamma globulin, if given early after exposure, may reduce the severity of the attack, but it is doubtful and may be unobtainable.

It is common for a cough to persist for several weeks after the onset, or to recur after a period of improvement. The possibility of partial collapse of the lung should be borne in mind in such cases, and when there is doubt a radiological examination is desirable.

The duration of infectivity is from two days before the start of the cough to five weeks after the start. Quarantine is not required.

The incubation period is 7–10 days.

References

ADASEK P.J., MEYER M.N. & RAY C.G. (1969) Antibiotic treatment of pertussis. *Pediatrics*, 44, 606.

ANON. (1969) Antibiotic treatment of pertussis (leading article). *Pediatrics*, 44, 474.

BASS J.W., KLENK E.L., KOTHEIMER J.B., LINNERMANN C.C. & SMITH, M.H.D. (1969) Antimicrobial treatment of pertussis. *J. Pediat.* 75, 768.

CONNOR J.D. (1970) Etiologic role of adenoviral infection in pertussis syndrome. *New Engl. J. Med.* 283, 390.

MEDICAL RESEARCH COUNCIL (1953) Treatment of whooping cough with antibiotics. *Lancet*, 1, 1109.

SHIRKEY H.C. (1968) *Pediatric Therapy 1968–1969.* St. Louis, Mosby.

WILMS' TUMOUR (Nephroblastoma)

This is a rare condition. If a child is suspected of having a Wilms' tumour, he should be referred to the hospital as an emergency.

Different regimes of treatment are in use, but the superiority of one over any other has not been established. The tumour will certainly be removed, completely if possible, followed by radiotherapy. The treatment is then likely to be continued with actinomycin D and vincristine – the latter particularly if there are metastases.

The discovery of a Wilms' tumour in an apparently well child is a devastating experience for a family, and the family doctor will need to be especially sensitive in his handling of the situation.

WIND

See *Infant Feeding*, p. 47.
See also *Sleep Problems*, p. 241.

WORMS

Roundworm

The treatment consists of bephenium or piperazine, without previous preparation given as follows:

Piperazine, 2–3 g. single dose.
or Bephenium (Alcopar)
age 1:   2·5 g. ⎫
age 5:   5 g.   ⎬   Single dose, in morning before food.
Puberty: 5 g.   ⎭

Tapeworm

For tapeworm the treatment is dichlorophen in a single dose of 70 mg./kilo in divided doses, without previous purgation or starvation; or niclosamide in the morning on an empty stomach. No solid food is given for two hours after the second dose; no purgation is necessary.

Mepacrine and filix mas are no longer recommended.

Dichlorophen (Antiphen) 500 mg. tablet.
age 1–5 years: 0·5–2 g. single dose
6–12 years: 2–4 g. single dose
or Niclosamide (Yomesan) 500 mg. tablets
age 1–5 years: 0·5 g.   } repeated one hour later in the
6–12 years: 0·5–1 g.   } morning before food without fasting.

Threadworms

Most school children have threadworms, and unless they are producing symptoms in the form of pruritus ani, no treatment is required.

The treatment of choice is either Viprynium or Piperazine. The Viprynium tablets should be swallowed whole to avoid staining the mouth, and the parents and child should be told that the stools will be stained red.

It used to be stated that if one child is treated for threadworms, the whole family should be treated, on the ground that everyone else in the house will also have been infected. It is now uncertain whether this is necessary.

Theoretically the infection would be cured if the child avoided reinfection by never touching food or putting his fingers in his mouth without prior washing of the hands. This is too much to expect.

Viprynium Embolate (Vanquin) 50 mg. tablets. Suspension 10 mg./ml.
age 1 year: 75 mg.   } Single dose.
7 years: 150 mg. } Second dose in 3 weeks.
Puberty: 300 mg. }

Piperazine – pripsen granules (containing senokot).
age up to 6 years: 7·5 g.
6 years and over: 10g.
Single dose, repeated in one week.

Ankylostoma

This infection is treated with Bephenium.

Appendixes

Appendixes

OFFICIAL AND TRADE NAMES OF DRUGS

Official name	Trade name
Acetazolamide	Diamox
Acetylcysteine	Airbron
Actinomycin D	Dactinomycin
Aluminium Hydroxide GEL	Aludrox
Amitriptyline	Tryptizol, Saroten, Laroxyl
Amphotericin B	Fungilin
Ampicillin	Penbritin
Atropine Methyl Nitrate	Eumydrin
Azathioprine	Imuran
Bacitracin Ointment with neomycin	Neobactrin
Beclomethazone	Propaderm
Benzalkonium	Drapolene, Calaxin, Roccal
Benzathine Penicillin	Penidural
Benzoic Acid Compound Ointment	Whitfield's Ointment (Official synonym)
Benzyl Penicillin	Solupen, Crystapen G
Benzyl Penicillin BP	Falopen
Benzyl Penicillin Potassium	Cathopen, Eskacillin
Benzyl Penicillin Sodium	Crystapen (Inj.)
Bephenium	Alcopar
Betamethazone with Chlortetracycline	Betnovate A
Betamethazone with Clioquinol	Betnovate C
Betamethazone Valerate	Betnovate
Bisacodyl	Dulcolax
Bromhexine Hydrochloride	Bisolvon
Brompheniramine Maleate	Dimotane
Carbamazepine	Tegretol
Carbenicillin	Pyopen
Carbenoxalone	Biogastrone
Cephalexin	Keflex, Ceporex
Cephaloridine	Ceporin
Cetrimide	Cetavlon
Chloramphenicol	Chloromycetin
Chlordiazepoxide	Librium
Chlorhexidine	Hibitane
Chlorpheniramine	Piriton
Chlorpromazine	Largactil
Chlortetracycline	Aureomycin
Choline Theophyllinate	Choledyl
Clindamycin	Dalacin C
Clioquinal	Enterovioform
Clomocycline	Megachlor

Official name	*Trade name*
Cloxacillin	Orbenin
Colistin	Colomycin
Corticotrophin	ACTH
Cyclopentolate	Cyclogyl, Mydrilate
Demethylchlortetracycline	Ledermycin
Dextromethorphan	Romilar
Diazepam	Valium
Dichlorophen	Antiphen
Dicophane	DDT (Official synonym)
Dicyclomine Hydrochloride	Merbentyl
Dimercaprol	BAL
Diphenhydramine	Benadryl
Diphenoxylate with atropine	Lomotil
Disodium Cromoglycate	Intal
Erythromycin	Erythrocin, Ilotycin, Ilosone
Ethamivan	Vandid
Ethosusuximide	Zarontin, Emeside
Fenfluramine	Ponderax
Ferrous Sulphate Co	Fersolate
Flufenamic Acid	Arlef 100
Flumethazone	Locorten
Flumethazone with Neomycin	Locorten N
Fluocinolone Acetonide	Synalar
Fluocinolone with Neomycin	Synalar N
Framycetin	Soframycin
Fusidic Acid or sodium fusidate	Fucidin
Gamma Benzene Hexachloride	Lorexane
Gentamicin	Genticin, Cidomycin
Hexachlophane	Phisohex, Disfex, Sterzac, Cidal, Gamoflen
Hydrocortisone with Neomycin	Neocortef
Hydrocortisone with Sodium Fusidate	Fucidin H
Ibuprofen	Brufen
Imipramine	Tofranil
Indomethacin	Indocid
Iron Dextran	Imferon
Isoniazid	INH
Kanamycin	Kantrex, Kanasyn
Lymecycline	Armyl, Mucomycin, Tetralysal

Official name	*Trade name*
Meclizine	Ancolan
Mepacrine	Atebrin
Meprobamate	Equanil, Miltown
Mepyramine	Anthisan
Methacycline	Rondomycin
Methandienone	Dianabol
Methdilazine	Dilosyn
Methicillin	Celbenin
Methylphenidate	Ritalin
Mexenone	Uvistat
Monosulphiram	Tetmosol
Nalidixic Acid	Negram
Nalorphine	Lethidrone
Neomycin	Neomin, Nivemycin
Neomycin Chlorhexidine Nasal Cream	Naseptin
Niclosamide	Yomesan
Nikethamide	Coramine
Nitrazepam	Mogadon
Nitrofurantoin	Furadantin, Berkfurin
Norethandrolone	Nilevar
Norethynodrel	Enavid
Novobiocin	Albamycin, Cathomycin
Nystatin with Hydrocortisone	Nystaform
Orciprenaline	Alupent
Oxytetracycline	Terramycin, Imperacin, Clinimycin
Paracetamol	Panadol, Tabalgin, Calpol, Cetal, Eneril, Febrilix
Pentobarbitone	Nembutal
Phenethicillin Potassium BP	Broxil
Pheneturide	Benuride
Phenindamine	Thephorin
Phenmetrazine	Preludin
Phenobarbitone	Luminal
Phenoxymethyl Penicillin	Penicillin V, Crystapen V, Distaquaine V, Pedipacs V Cil K, Penicals, Stabillin VK, Campocillin VK, V Cil K.
Phensuccimide	Milontin
Phenylazopyridine	Pyridium
Phenytoin	Epanutin
Phytomenadione (Vitamin K)	Konakion
Primidone	Mysoline
Procaine Penicillin	Distaquaine G, Prostabilin

Official name	*Trade name*
Procaine Penicillin with Benzyl Penicillin and Benethamine Penicillin	Triplopen
Prochlorperazine	Stemetil
Promethazine	Phenergan
Propantheline Bromide	Probanthine
Propicillin Potassium BP	Ultrapen, Brocillin
Quinalbarbitone	Seconal
Salbutamol	Ventolin
Sodium Calcium Edetate	EDTA
Succinyl Sulphathiazole	Sulfasuxidine
Sulphacetamide	Albucid
Sulphadimidine	Sulphamethazine
Sulphafurazole	Gantrisin
Sulphamethizole	Urolucosil
Sulphamethoxazole	Gantanol
Sulphamethoxypyridazine	Lederkyn, Midicel
Sulphaphenazole	Orisulf
Sulphasalazine	Salazopyrin
Sulphathiazole, Sulphadiazine, Sulphamerazine	Sulphatriad
Sulphathiazole, Sulphadiazine, Sulphadimidine with Streptomycin	Streptotriad
Sulthiame	Ospolot
Tetracosactrin	Synachthen
Tetracycline	Achromycin, Ambramycin, Tetracyn, Tetrex, Totomycin, Tetrachel, Steclin, Clititetrin
Tetracycline with Amphotericin	Mysteclin
Theophylline + Ephedrine + Phenobarbitone	Tedral, Franol
Thioridazine	Melleril
Tolnaftate	Tinaderm
Triamcinolone	Adcortyl
Triamcinolone Acetonide	Remiderm
Trimeprazine	Vallergan
Trimethoprim with Sulphamethoxazole	Septrin, Bactrim
Tropicamide	Mydriacyl
Troxidone	Tridione
Viprynium Embonate	Vanquin

Trade name	Official name
ACTH	Corticotrophin
Achromycin	Tetracycline
Adcortyl	Triamcinolone
Airbron	Acetylcysteine
Albamycin	Novobiocin
Albucid	Sulphacetamide
Alcopar	Bephenium
Aludrox	Aluminium Hydroxide GEL
Alupent	Orciprenaline
Ambramycin	Tetracycline
Ancolan	Meclizine
Anthisan	Mepyramine
Antiphen	Dichlorophen
Arlef 100	Flufenamic acid
Armyl	Lymecycline
Atebrin	Mepacrine
Aureomycin	Chlortetracycline
BAL	Dimercaprol
Bactrim	Trimethoprim with Sulphamethoxazole
Benadryl	Diphenhydramine
Benuride	Pheneturide
Berkfurin	Nitrofurantoin
Betnovate	Betamethazone Valerate
Betnovate A	Bethamethazone with Chlortetracycline
Betnovate C	Betamethazone with Clioquinol
Biogastrone	Carbenoxalone
Bisolvon	Bromhexidine Hydrochloride
Brocillin	Propicillin Potassium BP
Broxil	Phenethicillin Potassium BP
Brufen	Ibuprofen
Calaxin	Benazlkonium
Calpol	Paracetamol
Campocillin VK	Phenoxymethyl Penicillin
Cathomycin	Novobiocin
Cathopen	Benzyl Penicillin Potassium
Celbenin	Methicillin
Ceporex	Cephalexin
Ceporin	Cephaloridine
Cetal	Paracetamol
Cetavlon	Cetrimide
Chloromycetin	Chloramphenicol
Choledyl	Choline Theophyllinate
Cidal	Hexochlophane
Cidomycin	Gentamicin
Clinimycin	Oxytetracycline

Trade name	*Official name*
Clititetrin	Tetracycline
Colomycin	Colistin
Coramine	Nikethamide
Crystapen (Inj.)	Benzyl Penicillin Sodium
Crystapen G	Benzyl Penicillin
Crystapen V	Phenoxymethyl Penicillin
Cyclogyl	Cyclopentolate
DDT (Official synonym not trade name)	Dicophane
Dactinomycin	Actinomycin D
Dalacin C	Clindamycin
Diamox	Acetazolamide
Dianabol	Methandienone
Dilosyn	Methdilazine
Dimotane	Brompheniramine Maleate
Disfex	Hexochlophane
Distaquaine G	Procain Penicillin
Distaquaine V	Phenoxymethyl Penicillin
Drapolene	Benzalkonium
Dulcolax	Bisacodyl
EDTA	Sodium Calcium Edetate
Emeside	Ethosusuximide
Enavid	Norethynodrel
Eneril	Paracetamol
Enterovioform	Clioquinal
Epanutin	Phenytoin
Equanil	Meprobamate
Erythrocin	Erythromycin
Eskacillin	Benzyl Penicillin Potassium
Eumydrin	Atropine Methyl Nitrate
Falopen	Benzyl Penicillin BP
Febrilix	Paracetamol
Fersolate	Ferrous Sulphate Co
Franol	Theophylline+Ephedrine+ Phenobarbitone
Fucidin	Fusidic Acid or sodium fusidate
Fucidin H	Hydrocortisone with Sodium Fusidate
Fungilin	Amphotericin B
Furadantin	Nitrofurantoin
Gamoflen	Hexochlophane
Gantanol	Sulphamethoxazole
Gantrisin	Sulphafurazole
Genticin	Gentamycin
Hibitane	Chlorhexidine

Trade name	Official name
INH	Isoniazid
Ilosone	Erythromycin
Ilotycin	Erythromycin
Imferon	Iron Dextran
Imperacin	Oxytetracycline
Imuran	Azathioprine
Indocid	Indomethacin
Intal	Disodium Cromoglycate
Kanasyn	Kanamycin
Kantrex	Kanamycin
Keflex	Cephalexin
Konakion	Phytomenadione (Vitamin K)
Largactil	Chlorpromazine
Laroxyl	Amitriptyline
Lederkyn	Sulphamethoxypyridazine
Ledermycin	Demethylchlortetracycline
Lethidrone	Nalorphine
Librium	Chlordiazepoxide
Locorten	Flumethazone
Locorten N	Flumethazone with Neomycin
Lomotil	Diphenoxylate with atropine
Lorexane	Gamma Benzene Hexachloride
Luminal	Phenobarbitone
Megachlor	Clomocycline
Melleril	Thioridazine
Merbentyl	Dicyclomine Hydrochloride
Midicel	Sulphamethoxypyridazine
Milontin	Phensuximide
Miltown	Meprobamate
Mogadon	Nitrazepam
Mucomycin	Lymecycline
Mydriacyl	Tropicamide
Mydrilate	Cyclopentolate
Mysoline	Primidone
Mysteclin	Tetracycline with Amphotericin
Naseptin	Neomycin Chlorhexidine Nasal Cream
Negram	Nalidixic Acid
Nembutal	Pentobarbitone sodium
Neobactrin	Bacitracin Ointment with neomycin
Neocortef	Hydrocortisone with Neomycin
Neomin	Neomycin
Nilevar	Norethandrolone
Nivemycin	Neomycin

Trade name	*Official name*
Nystaform	Nystatin with Hydrocortisone
Orbenin	Cloxacillin
Orisulf	Sulphaphenazole
Ospolot	Sulthiame
Panadol	Paracetamol
Pedipacs V Cil K	Phenoxymethyl Penicillin
Penbritin	Ampicillin
Penicals	Phenoxymethyl Penicillin
Penicillin V	Phenoxymethyl Penicillin
Penidural	Benzathine Penicillin
Phenergan	Promethazine
Phisohex	Hexochlophane
Piriton	Chlorpheniramine
Ponderax	Fenfluramine
Preludin	Phenmetrazine
Probanthine	Propantheline Bromide
Propaderm	Beclomethazone
Prostabilin	Procaine Penicillin
Pyopen	Carbenicillin
Pyridium	Phenylazopyridine
Remidern	Triamcinolone Acetonide
Ritalin	Methylphenidate
Roccal	Benzalkonium
Romilar	Dextromethorphan
Rondomycin	Methacycline
Salazopyrin	Sulphasalazine
Saroten	Amitriptyline
Seconal	Quinalbarbitone
Septrin	Trimethoprim with Sulphamethoxazole
Soframycin	Framycetin
Solupen	Benzyl Penicillin
Stabillin VK	Phenoxymethyl Penicillin
Steclin	Tetracycline
Stemetil	Prochlorperazine
Sterzac	Hexochlophane
Streptotriad	Sulphathiazole, Sulphadiazine Sulphadimidine with Streptomycin
Sulfasuxidine	Succinyl Sulphathiazole
Sulphamethazine	Sulphadimidine
Sulphatriad	Sulphathiazole, Sulphadiazine, Sulphamerazine
Synachthen	Tetracosactrin
Synalar	Fluocinolone Acetonide

Trade name	*Official name*
Synalar N	Fluocinolone with Neomycin
Tabalgin	Paracetamol
Tedral	Theophylline+Ephedrine+ Phenobarbitone
Tegretol	Carbamazepine
Terramycin	Oxytetracycline
Tetmosol	Monosulphiram
Tetrachel	Tetracycline
Tetracyn	Tetracycline
Tetralysal	Lymecycline
Tetrex	Tetracycline
Thephorin	Phenindamine
Tinaderm	Tolnaftate
Tofranil	Imipramine
Totomycin	Tetracycline
Tridione	Troxidone
Triplopen	Procain Penicillin with Benzyl Penicillin and Benethamine Penicillin
Tryptizol	Amitriptyline
Ultrapen	Propicillin Potassium BP
Urolucosil	Sulphamethizole
Uvistat	Mexenone
V Cil K	Phenoxymethyl Penicillin
Valium	Diazepam
Vallergan	Trimeprazine
Vandid	Ethamivan
Vanquin	Viprynium Embonate
Ventolin	Salbutamol
Whitfield's Ointment (Official synonym not trade name)	Benzoic Acid Compound Ointment
Yomesan	Niclosamide
Zarontin	Ethosusuximide

MEAN WEIGHT OF CHILDREN

| | Boys | | | Girls | |
Age	Pounds	Kg		Pounds	Kg.
1	22	10		21	10
2	28	13		27	12
3	32	15		32	14
4	37	17		36	16
5	41	18		40	18
6	45	20		45	20
7	50	23		50	23
8	55	25		55	25
9	61	27		61	28
10	67	30		69	31

SOME EQUIVALENTS

Weight

15 grains (gr.) = 1 gramme (g.)	= 1,000 mg.
10	600 mg.
7½	450
5	300
4	250
3	200
2½	150
2	125
1½	100
1	60
¾	50
½	30
¼	15
1/10	6
1/12	5
1/20	3
1/25	2·5
1/50	1·25
1/60	1·0
1/75	0·8
1/100	0·6
1/150	0·4
1/200	0·3
1/500	0·125

1,000 microgrammes (µg.) = 1 mg.

$\frac{1}{4}$ oz. = 7 g.
$\frac{1}{2}$ oz. = 14 g.
$\frac{3}{4}$ oz. = 21 g.
1 oz. = 28 g.

1 lb. = 454 g.
1 kg. 2·3 lb.

Liquid measures

oz.	ml.
$\frac{1}{2}$	14
$\frac{3}{4}$	21
1	28
$1\frac{1}{2}$	42
$1\frac{3}{4}$	49
2	57
$2\frac{1}{2}$	71
3	85
4	113
5	142
6	170

1 ml. 15 minims
1 fluid drachm (dr.) = 4 ml. = 60 minims = 1 average teaspoon
1 pint 560 ml.
1·8 pints 1 litre
1 litre 35 fluid oz.

Temperature – Fahrenheit – Centigrade equivalents

Fahrenheit	Centigrade
86	30
87	30·6
88	31·1
89	31·7
90	32·2
91	32·7
92	33·3
93	33·8
94	34·4
95	35
96	35·5
97	36·1

Fahrenheit	Centigrade
98	36·6
99	37·2
100	37·7
101	38·3
102	38·8
103	39·4
104	40
105	40·5
106	41·1

Some Relevant and Recommended Books

APLEY J. & MACKEITH R. (1968) *The Child and his Symptoms.* Oxford, Blackwell Scientific Publications.

BECKMAN H. (1967) *Dilemmas in Drug Therapy.* Philadelphia, Saunders.

ELLIS M. (1967) *Accidents to Children.* London, Evans Brothers.

GELLIS S.S. & KAGAN B.M. (1970) *Current Pediatric Therapy.* Philadelphia, Saunders.

ILLINGWORTH R.S. (1964) *The Normal School Child.* London, Heinemann Medical Books.

ILLINGWORTH R.S. (1968) *The Normal Child.* 4th edn. London, Churchill.

ILLINGWORTH R.S. (1971) *Common Symptoms of Disease in Children.* 3rd edn. Oxford, Blackwell Scientific Publications.

JONES P.G. (1970) *Clinical Paediatric Surgery.* Bristol, Wright.

MATTHEW H. & LAWSON A.A.H. (1967) *Treatment of Common Acute Poisonings.* Edinburgh, Livingstone.

MEYLER L. & PECK H.M. (1968) *Drug Induced Diseases.* Excerpta Medica Foundation.

NIXON H.H. & O'DONNELL B. (1966) *The Essentials of Paediatric Surgery,* 2nd edn. London, Heinemann Medical Books.

ROOK A., WILKINSON D.S. & EBLING F.J.G. (1968) *Textbook of Dermatology.* Oxford, Blackwell Scientific Publications.

SHARRARD W. J. W. (1971) *Paediatric Orthopaedics and Fractures.* Oxford, Blackwell Scientific Publications.

SHIRKEY H.C. (1968) *Pediatric Therapy 1968–1969.* St. Louis, Mosby.

SNEDDON I.B. & CHURCH R.E. (1964) *Practical Dermatology.* London, Arnold.

WADE O. L. (1971) Adverse reactions to drugs. London, Heinemann.

Some Relevant and Recommended Books

Index